The Story of the Minnesota Influence on American Surgery

Table of Contents

Preface
Reflections: On Dr. Owen H. Wangensteen

Chapter 1
Dr. Owen H. Wangensteen – Department History and Academic Approach

Chapter 2
Personal Observations by Dr. Wangensteen's Staff Assistant, Mildred Jones

Chapter 3
Dr. Lester Dragstedt Interview
Dr. Wangensteen's Contributions in Intestinal Obstruction, Ulcer Physiology, Cancer, and his Fundamental Approach to Resident Training

Chapter 4
The Ulcer Story

Chapter 5
The Cancer Detection Center

Chapter 6
The Heart Story

Chapter 7
The Impact of Earl Bakken and his Associates on Cardiology and Cardiac Surgery (Dr. C. Walton Lillehei) – Coordination of Industry and Medicine

*To my wife Mary,
for her 60 years of
support and love.*

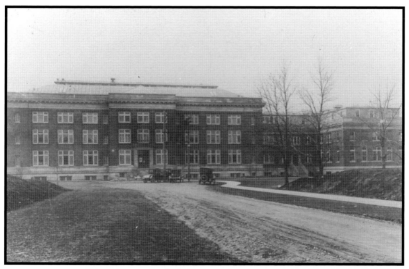

The University of Minnesota Hospital in the 1930's

Through The Portals of Pigs and Manure

Preface

Reflections: On Owen H. Wangensteen

In interviews over the years with several of the trainees who became department or division heads (37 in all), their experiences in the Wangensteen program were similar. Once they were interviewed by Dr. Wangensteen and then offered a resident position in the Department of Surgery at the University of Minnesota, there was a deep sense of gratitude and all offered special affection for the "Chief." It was quickly understood that hard work, sharing ideas, diligence in patient care, completing laboratory tasks and presenting problems for critical analysis at weekly conferences was expected. Laboratory experience, as suggested by Dr. Wangensteen, was essential for learning surgical technique and it most importantly stimulates one's mind to creativity in attempts to solve basic problems in the surgical arena. Even if Dr. Wangensteen had the idea initially, the individual effort by his residents to bring the problem to fruition was rewarded by a trip to what was called the Surgical Forum at the American College of Surgeons, to present the research to the great surgical teachers of the time. All were thus bitten by their surgical achievements and thus were convinced to stay in the surgical area as academicians.

A basic science education such as physiology and the like all paved the way to problem solving in the Wangensteen program. The enthusiasm generated in this learned atmosphere affected all of their lives forever and prepared them for their own head positions. Dr. Wangensteen himself was the catalyst and became engrossed in full detail in most of the experimental designs. Moreover, Dr. Wangensteen's elephantine memory, exemplified by his grasp of history and references of the basic problem at hand, was indeed stimulating. His ability to stimulate the younger generation and provide an atmosphere of intellectual competitiveness as well as friendly learning was the basis of his program. He fashioned himself as a Gunga Din, the regimental water carrier. Also, the coordination of basic science added to his program. The provocative basic science conferences with professors all added up to great progress in fields which at the time were yet untested. Because of the ambiance in research with Dr. Wangensteen setting the example, fledgling officers became enthralled with basics far beyond technical surgical skills and welcomed time spent in the laboratory. Many individuals spent prolonged time in basic programs such as immunology, biophysics, and physiology to gain their basic graduate degrees.

Dr. Wangensteen wholeheartedly supported his trainees no matter where they went. He visited them, provided advice and acted, in many instances, like a surrogate father. Even when mistakes were made, he would somehow turn adversity into advantage. Dr. Wangensteen's program was meant to tap restless intelligence in surgical fledglings to discover better ways to treat problems. In his own words, "To give accelerated momentum to the enlargement of knowledge, the capacity to dream and share with one's associates; these were the ingredients of inspired research."

As Henry Adams said, "A teacher affects eternity. He can never tell where his influence stops." Of all his accomplishments including his original work in intestinal obstruction and decompression drainage, surgical concepts in treatment of gastric and duodenal ulcers, and his monumental support of the cardiac surgery and the cancer detection program, Dr. Wangensteen's legacy for the Minnesota influence on American surgery remains his catalytic influence on young house officers stimulating them to an academic surgery career. Opportunity was the paymaster.

Chapter 1

Owen H. Wangensteen – Department History and Academic Approach

Dr. Owen Wangensteen (1898-1981), distinguished professor of surgery and head of the Department of Surgery at the University of Minnesota from 1930 to 1967 was a superb teacher, courageous scientist, imaginative surgeon, generous advisor, and a very noble man. He had tremendous faith in young people and in the University as a concept. He also had a great deal of respect for the library and found it to be a great source of scientific truth. He believed history repeated itself in many ways, and was responsible for many of the present basic surgical principles and techniques. Modern influences improved and changed many of these early attempts to solve medical problems. Most importantly, he believed in the virtue of change. He had an inexhaustible supply of energy, and greatly influenced all he touched.

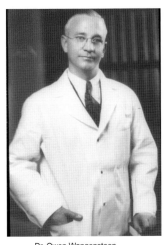
Dr. Owen Wangensteen

His confidence in young people was impregnable and he was a surrogate father to many of us in the program. He will go down in history as one of the great surgical teachers, if not the greatest in the 20th century. It would be redundant in the next several pages to aggrandize Dr. Wangensteen for his numerous accomplishments; president of numerous surgical associations including the American College of Surgeons and the prestigious American Surgical Association, his numerous honorary degrees and medals, and some 870 publications and books and editor of the Journal of Surgery. Rather, you should understand the development of Dr. Wangensteen's career and how he influenced his surgical school and his medical contemporaries in the field of American surgery. His numerous scientific accomplishments as an educator were dwarfed by his catalytic influence on young house officers by displaying his ability to spark enthusiasm and tap the resources of their potential creativity. This is the essence of his accomplishments and will serve as his remembrance for tomorrow. Moreover, his alliance with other departments such as Dr. Maurice Visscher's Department of Physiology, and Dr. Jesse Edwards in Cardiac Pathology, were very important in the development of his residents as they provided coordinated stimulation to his graduate program.

Now, how did Dr. Wangensteen enter into the field of medicine? He was born in Lake Park, Minnesota on September 21, 1898, where he was raised on a farm. He actually felt a mysterious charm in that occupation. He enjoyed nature and nurturing plants and animals. One spring when he was in

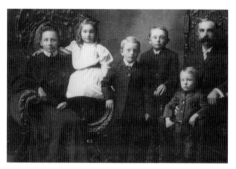

OHW in his youth

high school, there were a number of Poland sows sired by Yorkshire boars that were sickly and could not farrow their young. His father called a veterinarian to the farm who suggested that because of a nutritional problem, the sows be sent to slaughter in South St. Paul. However, Owen, who was devoted and very interested in the sows asked his father if he could try to save them. His father had previously purchased an apparatus, through an advertising column in a farm journal, for delivering piglets. However, in this instance, the apparatus proved impractical. Owen then began delivering the piglets by hand. Although the effort took approximately three weeks, he delivered 300 piglets and salvaged all but two of the sows.

Through The Portals of Pigs and Manure

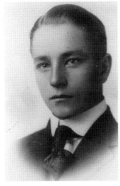
OHW as a late teenager

To say the least, young Owen was greatly influenced by this accomplishment. In addition his father wanted nothing more than for Owen to become a physician. However, at that time, young Owen wanted to become a veterinarian, influenced by his love for the farm. In either instance, he knew he would need basic education. He applied to the University of Minnesota, was accepted, and spent three years in the Science Literature and Arts programs. During summer vacations, Owen had to work on the farm in order to help pay for his education. He went home and sure enough, there was a tremendous amount of haying and hauling of manure to be done. This endeavor became a very arduous task. Finally, at the end of one hot summer day, after he had handled a great deal of manure in exceptional heat, he decided that a professional career in medicine would be his future choice. Again his father confronted him regarding the thought of becoming a physician and at this time, young Owen capitulated. Dr. Wangensteen often told me, and to others, that it was through portals of pigs and manure that he decided to go into the medical field.

OHW as a pre-med student

As a pre-medical student, Owen did very well in school. He entered medical school after SLA, and graduated in 1922 as a Doctor of Medicine with honors at the top of his class. Owen heard a lecture when he was a junior medical student by Dr. Arthur Strachauer (who at that time was Wangensteen's predecessor as Chairman of the Department of Surgery). He was greatly stimulated to the point that he felt surgery would be for him, the most dramatic area of medicine. As he stated, "That's where the action is." He certainly proved that throughout his illustrious career.

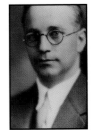
OHW in medical school

The Story of the Minnesota Influence on American Surgery

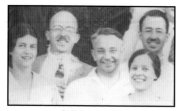
OHW as an intern

Although Dr. Wangensteen wanted to go into surgery right away, there were no fellowships available in the Department of Surgery. He decided, therefore, to accept one in the Department of Medicine as a preliminary step to surgery. The yearly stipend was only $600 and he was told he would have to work in a research laboratory. Reluctantly he was forced into research. But, as he demonstrated later in life, he discovered not only was this a very stimulating area, it became the basis for his future philosophies and activities.

Following that year in research in 1924, he spent a year at the Mayo Clinic in Rochester, Minnesota. At that time, Dr. Will Mayo observed his brilliant mind, elephantine memory and clinical acumen. Dr. Mayo was a great influence on Dr. Wangensteen, especially in the basic workings of the Mayo Clinic. When Dr. Wangensteen returned in January of 1925 to the University of Minnesota, he

Dr. Will Mayo

entered into the laboratory as a graduate fellow, and completed work on a Doctorate of Philosophy in surgery. He worked on the problem of undescended testes and did a superb job. During his Ph.D. exam,

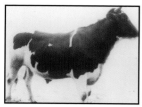
Ph.D.. Thesis: Undescended Testes

one of his classmates, Larry Larsen, said that when Owen took his Ph.D. exam, the examiners finally gave up because they could not ask him any questions he could not answer.

After finishing his fellowship, Owen was offered a job elsewhere at $15,000 a year. Despite the much higher salary, he refused the position because he wanted to stay at the University of Minnesota. Why? The charisma of the University and its vast potential for research and development were important in his decision. Prior to that period of time at the University, there had been a group of mediocre colleges that were run by rather dormant, self-satisfying individuals. When George Vincent became president of the University, he appointed Dr.

11

Through The Portals of Pigs and Manure

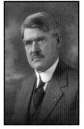
Dr. Elias Lyon

Elias Lyon as dean of the medical school. This was a brilliant decision. Dean Lyon became a tremendous influence on Owen Wangensteen and the school of medicine. By exercising his power of appointment, Dr. Lyon made full-time academic appointments in key medical school positions, surgery being one of them. Prior to that time, department heads worked part-time. The individuals appointed had great dedication towards graduate school education and improved the surroundings and atmosphere in the University School of Medicine. Within a period of 6 short years, under the influence of President Vincent and Dean Lyon, the University became a vibrant thriving complex. The spirit of research and graduate education kindled many fires. As Drs. Daniel Gillman, Henry William Welch and Bradshaw Brown had influenced plans of eastern education, President George Vincent and Dean Elias Lyon stimulated the University of Minnesota Medical School into a first rate institution.

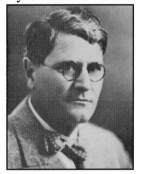
Dr. Strachauer

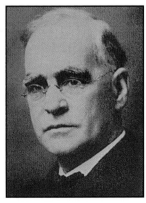
Dr. James Moore

Dr. James Moore, once a private practitioner, became the first full-time surgery head. This was due to a medical problem that forced him to give up the rigors of private practice. He was dedicated to his full-time position as head of surgery prior to Dr. Strachauer's tenure in the position. They both influenced educational trends by instituting graduate degrees in clinical sciences. They were both responsible for a strong alliance with the Mayo Clinic. These men were the ones who stimulated Dr. Wangensteen's decision to stay at the University.

A search committee for a new chairman of the Department of Surgery was formed in 1926 because Dr. Strachauer, the current chairman at the time was about to retire. The search committee called in a number of candidates, including Dr. Francis Newton of Harvard and Dr. Mont Reid of Cincinnati. Both had completed their training at John Hopkins under the tutorage of Dr. William Halsted, the famous Professor of Surgery. Professor Halsted at the time was the leading

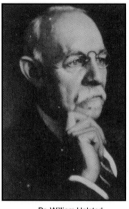 surgical professor and influenced a number of training programs during that period. The search committee interviewed both individuals and both candidates inspected the Department of Surgery at the University of Minnesota. Dr. Newton and Dr. Reid both said there was nothing of value at the University nor would there ever be. They both declined the Department of Surgery chairman position.

Dr. William Halsted

Meanwhile, Dean Elias Lyon and Dr. William Mayo were watching the brilliant progress of Dr. Wangensteen throughout his career at the University and the Mayo Clinic from 1915-1926. An administrative committee decided that Dr. Wangensteen, despite his young age of thirty years should be appointed as chairman of the Department of Surgery. Dr. Wangensteen expressed this was probably by default, however, he was very excited at the opportunity. He stated that, at that time, there were not many impressive buildings and funds were very scarce, in fact delinquent. There was a certain atmosphere the visitors of the department had overlooked. This was the scientific atmosphere created by Dean Elias Lyon, President George Vincent, Dr. James Moore, and Dr. Strachauer which had a great influence on Dr. Wangensteen's decision to take over the department.

Through The Portals of Pigs and Manure

Although Dr. Wangensteen was to be appointed chairman of the Department of Surgery, Dean Lyon, Dr. Mayo and Dr. Wangensteen's above contemporaries felt he would benefit from studying abroad with some of the great European surgical professors and teachers. In fact, Dr. Strachauer was kind enough to delay his retirement for four to five years until Dr. Wangensteen assumed the full chair in 1930. Before assuming this chair, and with the help of Dr. George Fahr, originally from Switzerland, who was an internist and cardiologist

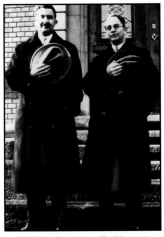

Dr. Fritz deQuervain and Dr. Wangensteen

at the General Hospital of Minneapolis (now Hennepin County Medical Center), it was arranged for Owen to visit Professor Asher in Berne and Fritz deQuervain, Dr. Theodore Kocher's pupil. He could to evaluate their careers and departments. These were great men of the time in the field of surgery. Clinically Dr. Wangensteen was very impressed with these individuals. He was disappointed, however in the lack of research at their institutions. He noticed that house officers became dissuaded from research because they were always given secondary tasks in the clinical arena, which consumed most of their time. The trainees of these men, however, became excellent clinical surgeons, the hallmark of these great European schools.

Dr. William Halsted of the John Hopkins program was one of the great surgical teachers at the time, and had a great influence on surgery throughout the United States and abroad. The Hopkins program required eight years beyond internship. These individuals however, spent most of their time in clinical endeavors, much as the European graduates. The house officers became very skilled and clinically versatile, and became specialized individuals in their surgical fields. In the Halsted program, however, minimal research had been carried out in the laboratory. After his trip abroad, Dr. Wangensteen began to plan his unique approach to surgical training. He was influenced by Dr. John Hunter, a great physiologist who

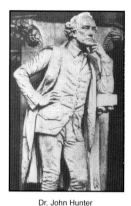

Dr. John Hunter

introduced the scientific approach to basic problems. Dr. Wangensteen closely studied his introduction of the scientific approach and eventually applied this concept to the field of surgery to improve clinical concepts.

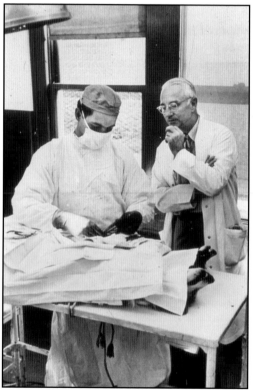

Dr. Wangensteen and Resident Raffuci

These individuals therefore were the ones who really stimulated Dr. Wangensteen to develop a very different type of surgery program. He felt individuals should spend one to three years in the laboratory devoted full-time to their research endeavors. Not only could surgical skills be learned, but their ideas could be tested and latent creativity and talent could be developed. Dr. Wangensteen influenced and supported their ideas. As stated, he had great faith in young minds and he was a rigorous taskmaster. The residents were rewarded with graduate degrees upon solving basic problems. This program became the basis for his success and was responsible for his numerous accomplishments in the surgical field. He started the University of Minnesota program in 1930 with one surgical fellow and two interns and a little over 100

15

surgical beds. At his retirement in 1967, there were 100 surgical fellows, 18 interns and approximately the same amount of beds. He trained over 37 department or division heads and placed them in positions

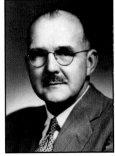

throughout the country. In his original program, over half of these individuals were spending at least two to three years in the laboratory. This research tradition was also maintained under the direction of Dr. John Najarian; Dr. Wangensteen's replacement at his retirement in 1967.

Dr. Maurice Visscher

One of the most important influences in the basic research program was Dr. Wangensteen's alliance with Dr. Maurice Visscher, the head of the Department of Physiology in 1936. He and Dr. Wangensteen became close friends. Dr. Wangensteen respected Dr. Visscher's work in the field of physiology, especially cardiology, the field he had been working on at the University of Chicago. This alliance was responsible for the advent of open-heart surgery at the University of Minnesota, the United States and around the world.

The interdisciplinary approach where intellectual individuals from several basic areas would get together weekly to discuss problems and criticize residents' ideas and experimental designs has remained the basis and the greatness whereby this school has achieved so many advancements in several areas including cardiac surgery.

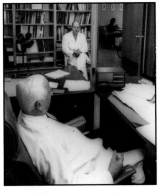

OHW discussing lab problems
with Dr. Bernstein

The key to Dr. Wangensteen's program was his flexibility. There was no systematic plan, as there had been clinically in the eastern schools, under the Halsted influence. Many individuals in the Minnesota program were motivated by their particular research program to spend at least two to three years in the laboratory. Growth, maturity and enthusiasm were kindled through this program. Across the country, for many years, it was frequently stated by many of the surgical educators at meetings that when residents entered Dr. Wangensteen's program, they would go through a tunnel and emerge as accomplished academic surgeons. What happened in that tunnel was a mystery to many of these individuals. Crawling through the tunnel, was a long and arduous task. Some individuals seemed to never emerge from that tunnel. Dr. Wangensteen never turned down a "good idea." He always found funds and graciously supported his residents.

Thus, the Wangensteen approach to develop independent researchers was to work toward a goal of graduate degrees and develop surgical skills in the laboratory. This was the essence of the Wangensteen surgical program. This became the basis of Wangensteen's training for nearly thirty seven full-time professors and division heads and over 100 fellows in other academic positions throughout the country. Dr. Wangensteen was also responsible for 12 Markle scholars (one of the most prestigious honors in academia). He often likened himself to Gunga Din, the regimental water carrier, as he influenced his students.

When individuals finished their complete training program, Dr. Wangensteen, in his own inimitable way, would pick up the phone and depending on the openings available at the time, place

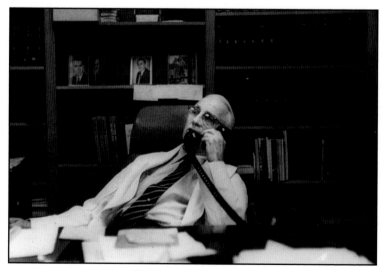

OHW placing an academic surgeon

these individuals in key surgical positions throughout the country He provided the suitcase when the position was obtained. He felt opportunity was the paymaster for continuing surgical education. He also stated that vibrant stimulating professors and teachers must communicate enthusiasm to their students and the students must, in turn, take a position and become independent.

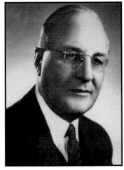

Dr. Evarts Graham

Emanating from his own research program, Dr. Wangensteen was also a great influence on the American College of Surgeons. In a letter to Dr. Evarts Graham, then president, he suggested what he called the Surgical Forum. This activity was predicated on his own meetings with scientists and professors who would meet weekly to discuss residents' research, and thus be constructively criticized by their peers. This activity provided an arena where young surgical fledglings, in programs throughout the country, could present their research, and be constructively criticized by surgery colleagues and professors. This yearly forum at the American College of Surgery meeting became a hallmark of surgical education, providing research stimulus to the surgical fledgling house officers throughout the country. Dr. Evarts Graham, then President of the American College of Surgeons, promoted the idea and program, and the first surgical forum was installed in the 1941 American College of Surgeons meeting. Fifty years later, a celebration of surgical research at the American College of Surgeons resulted in the dedication of the Surgical Forum to Dr. Owen H. Wangensteen.

How did Dr. Wangensteen support his rapidly growing department? In 1930, there was a department stipend of $30,000 given to him by the medical school. This was reduced to $20,000 in the following year because of the depression. This budget was far too small to support his ambitious endeavors. Thus, he decided to eradicate the stipends that were given to the part-time downtown clinical surgical teachers who taught in the Department of Surgery, and to those who

Through The Portals of Pigs and Manure

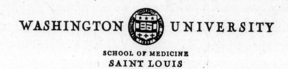

WASHINGTON 🏛 UNIVERSITY

SCHOOL OF MEDICINE
SAINT LOUIS

DEPARTMENT OF SURGERY
BARNES HOSPITAL
600 SOUTH KINGSHIGHWAY

February 7, 1941.

Dear Owen:

Your letter of February 3 concerning the proposed forum for the young surgeons has just reached me. I think it is a splendid idea to initiate this idea at the meeting at Minneapolis. I am also much interested in the program which you have arranged. It seems to me to be a very satisfactory one.

Your suggestion about writing to the professors of surgery informing them of the general plan and suggesting names of persons to contribute to the meeting to be held in Boston next fall also seems to me to be an excellent idea. I hope you will go ahead with it.

I wish the College had done something about this matter a few years ago. I am a little afraid that perhaps it is now too late to get the real value from it because of the recent organization of new societies based on the same general principle. I refer particularly, of course, to the Association of University Surgeons and, also, to the new Central States

Letter from Dr. Evarts Graham to OHW
regarding the surgical forum

19

took time away from their own private practices. By doing this, the extra money created allowed for Dr. Wangensteen to create six new research fellowship positions.

At the time this action was questioned by the new Dean Scammon and engendered quite a furor with the part-time clinical teachers whose salaries were cut. Thus, three years after Dr. Wangensteen had taken over the department, he received a phone call from Dean Scammon stating his surgery head position was in jeopardy because of this action. Dr. Wangensteen wrote a letter to the Dean and to the University of Minnesota's President, Lotus Coffman. He wrote that unless he was given full support, he would resign his position as department head and he would not return. He stated he would either be evicted, or accepted. He remained distant from the hospital for three weeks, spending much of this time contemplating the problem of intestinal obstruction. He began his first formulations of the virtue of intestinal suction for all forms of intestinal obstruction. These thoughts led to his investigations of the physiology of intestinal obstruction in the laboratory and the use of gastric suction to treat and help prevent its occurrence. This solution to the obstruction problem became one of his greatest accomplishments. These studies led to his first publication on obstruction, which was entered into an obscure Wisconsin journal in 1931 because the paper was turned down by some major surgical journals of the time. After this dormant period of three weeks, Dr. Wangensteen was finally given a vote of confidence from Dean Scammon and the key individuals who were responsible for the medical school. He was informed by the president's office that former Dean Lyon, Dr. Strachauer, Regent William J Mayo, and President Coffman gave him full support. Thus, he began his illustrious career and continued in the Department of Surgery as Chairman.

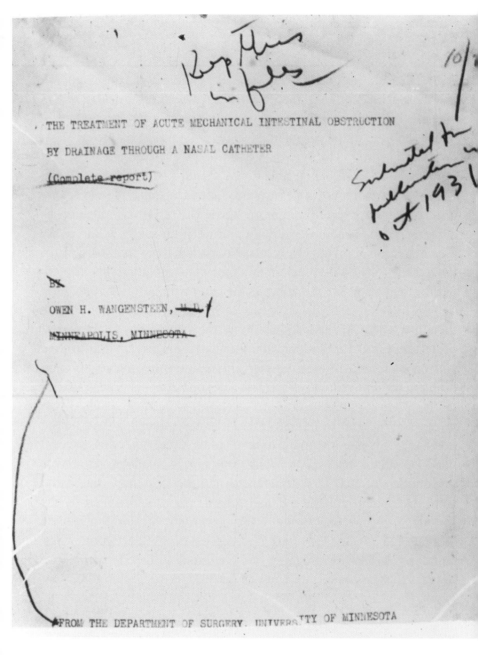

First Medical Journal (Wisconsin) to accept intestinal obstruction article

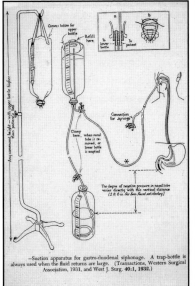

—Suction apparatus for gastro-duodenal siphonage. A trap-bottle is always used when the fluid returns are large. (Transactions, Western Surgical Association, 1931, and West J. Surg. 40:1, 1932.)

First intestinal obstruction device

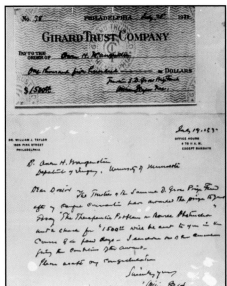

OHW Gross Prize

The rest of the monetary support over the years was stemmed from research grants generated by various activities from his residents and himself. Other support came from individuals who were affluent at the time. He would not send bills to individuals that he had operated on. Instead he told them he would appreciate a contribution to his department and his research fund. Individuals he knew, including the heads of various companies in Minnesota such as William McKnight, Chairman of Minnesota Mining and Manufacturing; David Paper, Chairman of Paper Calmensen; Frederick Weyerhaeuser, Chairman of Frederick Weyerhaeuser Lumber; John Pillsbury, CEO of Pillsbury; and so forth. Instead of giving them a bill for the amount he normally would charge for a procedure, these individuals were asked to contribute to his research fund. Thus, they contributed much greater funds to help support the department.

Also, of great importance to add to his financial support were his research luncheons, where residents would present their research to Dr. Wangensteen's friends and other affluent patrons. These luncheons stimulated a great number of contributions. He went before the state legislature to acquire funds for his department. At his retirement, it was estimated he had raised more than 10 million dollars for the University and the Department of Surgery, which was quite a significant amount of money at the time.

Then, he had the funds and the influence to provide the background for the stimulus of the many individuals who made great significant contributions in the surgical arena. Major breakthroughs occurred in various disciplines, and these were all generated by basic research in the laboratory. In the field of intestinal obstruction he devised a suction apparatus, which had a tremendous influence in the field of medicine. Dr. Maurice Visscher stated that by 1944, over 100,000 lives were saved by the Wangensteen suction. Ogden Nash wrote after surgery for his own intestinal obstruction, "May I find my final resting place in Owen Wangensteen's intestine, knowing that his mastery suction will assure me resurrection." For this accomplishment, Dr. Wangensteen received the John Scott Medal. This remained one of Minnesota's great influences on American surgery and medicine.

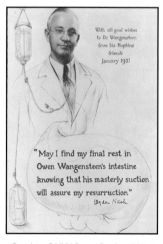

Card to OHW from Ogden Nash

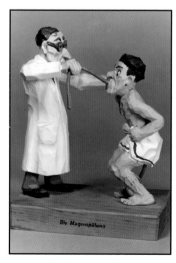

Die Magenspuluna

Through The Portals of Pigs and Manure

One of the greatest accomplishments of the 20th century was in the area of open-heart surgery. Why should cardiac surgery begin at the University of Minnesota and what was the influence of Dr. Maurice Visscher who was a cardiac physiologist and head of the Physiology Department? Among the number of individuals who had returned from the war in the 1940's was Dr. Clarence Dennis. He studied a system of bypassing the heart to oxygenate the body by mechanical means and he devised a rotating disc type of pump oxygenator under the aegis of Dr. Visscher

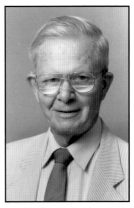

Dr. Clarence Dennis

and was fully supported by Dr. Wangensteen. Dr. Gibbon, from Philadelphia, had already worked on a membrane type oxygenator. At the time, there was a great need for some type of heart support so complex surgical operations could be carried out. Also, the method of bypassing the lungs and oxygenating the patients by these oxygenators had failed in human attempts. Dr. F. John Lewis had also returned from the war and elected to study hypothermia and its affect on cardiac physiology in the experimental laboratory. In addition, when Dr. C. Walton Lillehei returned from service, he worked on various aspects of cardiac physiology under the aegis of Dr. Maurice Visscher. Dr. Richard Varco nurtured many of these early individuals and provided excellent intellectual support, as did Dr. Wangensteen.

Incidentally, when Drs. F. John Lewis and Walt Lillehei came back from the service, both went to see Mrs. Jacobson who was Dr. Wangensteen's secretary at the time. She essentially ran the mechanics of the Department of Surgery at the University of Minnesota and told them to see Dr. Varco who was the executive officer in the department. Dr. Varco had told them there was not enough money to appoint any more residents. This was disappointing to Mrs. Jacobson so she suggested they see Dr. Wangensteen in person. At this meeting, Dr. C. Walton Lillehei discussed several new ideas regarding cardiac surgery, and immediately Dr. Wangensteen suggested he should start his fellowship. Dr. Wangensteen made the same suggestion to Dr. F. John Lewis and he found funds for both Dr. Lillehei and Dr. Lewis. This same type of event happened time and time again. Dr. Wangensteen never turned down a stimulating potential student and somehow, he always managed to acquire funds. The background was fertile for cardiac surgery with the alliance of the Department of Surgery, the Department of Physiology, the surgical laboratories, and the Wangensteen influence.

Just as the investigational programs were not by chance present in other fields, such as intestinal obstruction, or where Dr. Wangensteen proposed the beginning of a cancer detection programs in 1948, the field of cardiac surgery had its early origin. The first open-heart surgery was accomplished at the University of Minnesota under hypothermia by Dr. F. John Lewis and Dr. Varco in September of 1952. This accomplishment was predicated on Dr. F. John Lewis' work in the laboratory studying hypothermia and supported by Dr. Wangensteen and influenced by Dr. Maurice Visscher. Following this procedure, it was understood that when this surgery was carried out, there was a need for a heart/lung bypass and oxygenator to give more time for surgical correction of complex defects. Hypothermia gave only a limited intracardiac surgery period of five to seven minutes. In this first case, the large vessels to the heart, the superior venacava above and the inferior cava below were clamped, the heart upper chamber atrium was opened, and a simple interatrial septal defect (in the upper chamber of the heart) was observed. Fortunately, this was a simple defect and could be closed surgically within a few minutes under cooling of the body by hypothermia so the brain and organs

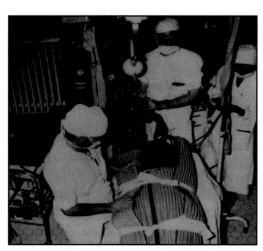

First open heart surgery under hypothermia

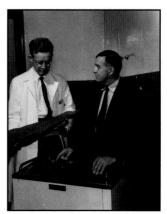

Dr. John Lewis and Dr. Richard Varco and cooling machine for first open heart surgery

would be preserved. This surgery was understood by all and acclaimed as the first open-heart procedure in the world. Even though this was a great accomplishment as the first open-heart operation to be performed, much further research and development in the preservation of circulation would have to be carried

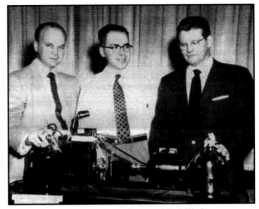

Drs. Walt Lillehei, Morley Cohen and Herb Warden
Cross Circulation Pump

out in order to correct much more complex congenital heart defects which included valve involvement and combined defects in the ventricular area. Dr. Wangensteen deserves a great deal of credit for supporting his researchers and stimulating them to greater accomplishments.

A great deal of research was then stimulated under the aegis of Dr. Maurice Visscher, the cardiac physiologist. Dr. Lillehei, Dr. Herbert Warden and Dr. Morley Cohen designed a bypass of the heart and lungs using live donor dogs and eventually humans as the donors. In 1954, the first operation was carried out by cross circulation where the heart defect patient's parent would act as the oxygenator. Dr. C. Walt Lillehei, Dr. Herbert Warden and Dr. Morley Cohen were the investigators for this accomplishment (see chapter 4 for details). This is another example of the Wangensteen approach where experiments in the laboratory provided the background for this surgery using cross circulation where two animals and a pump between them was used to keep the blood exchange between the dog patient and donor equal. One needed a 5:1 ratio in weight to gain equality of circulation. There was no oxygenator at this time.

Clinically, a "blue baby" arrived that was going to die, under Dr. Walt Lillehei and Dr. Richard Varco's care. Dr. Lillehei sent a note to Dr. Wangensteen asking him for permission to go ahead with cross circulation in the human. Dr. Wangensteen wrote back, "By all means, Walt, go ahead. Good luck." No committees, no fuss, no equivocations, despite objections from many of the clinical staff. In fact, it created a furor among many of the cardiologist internists and pediatricians that a research project was immediately carried out on a human being. In today's world, this would be a real problem because things are done by committee and one has to have FDA approval for these procedures. As Walt said at the time, "No wonder things got done around here." From the lab to the OR with the Wangensteen philosophy, the first complicated interventricular septum defect (tetrology of Fallot) was corrected through open-heart surgery. From that time, many firsts in cardiac surgery were performed using the cross circulation approach. With Dr. Wangensteen's influence, it was then recognized that because of some mistakes in cross circulation which will be discussed later, a pump oxygenator was necessary and had to be developed.

At that time, Dr. Richard Dewall, from Anoka, had been in general practice and wanted to go into surgery. He had heard of the Wangensteen program, and wanted to come and work in Dr. Wangensteen's laboratory. He was aware of the cross circulation technique but was interested in a new pump oxygenator and design. He came to see Dr. Wangensteen who suggested he apply to the graduate school for a research position in the Department of Surgery. He did apply, but was turned down by Dr. Blegan, then head of graduate school education, because his grades were not up to par (he was 111 of 177 in his medical school class and needed to be in the upper 25% for admission). Typical of Dr. Wangensteen, he found funds for Dr. Dick Dewall and hired him as a deaner in the lab, an animal attendant, rather than a part of the graduate program. In doing so, with the help and advice of Dr. Visscher, Dr. Dick Dewall worked out the physiology of a bubble type oxygenator and used a plastic helix and silicone to decrease the infused oxygen bubbles. The bubble oxygenator was thus developed. This was one of the great accomplishments in the laboratory and turned out to be the main device used for the correction of complicated open-heart surgery at the University of Minnesota and throughout the world. Dr. Dewall was under the Wangensteen program and he alone, was responsible for the salvage of thousands of lives undergoing complex congenital defect surgery, replacement of surgical valves and heart bypass for several operations on large vessels.

Through The Portals of Pigs and Manure

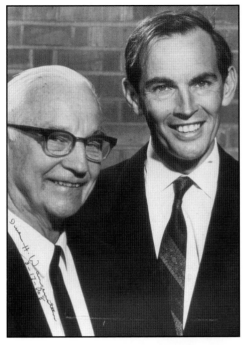

OHW and Dr. Christiaan Barnard

Also using this approach, Dr. Christiaan Barnard entered into the field of open-heart surgery by working in Dr. Wangensteen's lab learning experimental techniques. He also studied under Dr. Lillehei. Moreover, as he matured, he took lessons from Dr. Norman Shumway's original work in heart transplantation in animals. Dr. Barnard visited Dr. Shumway in California where he headed the cardiac program and visited Dr. Lawler in West Virginia. Christiaan Barnard performed the first heart transplant in summer of 1967 in Cape Town, South Africa. This was followed shortly thereafter by the first American heart transplant by Dr. Norman Shumway. It should be pointed out there was a great deal of frustration in this period regarding the first heart transplantation by Christiaan Barnard. Dr. Barnard had trained in the laboratory under Dr. Wangensteen and

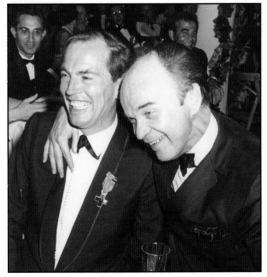

Dr. Barnard and Dr. Lillehei

then in Dr. Lillehei's lab to learn pump oxygenation techniques and was to return to South Africa. He had no funds and no equipment, so Dr. Wangensteen obtained funds and through the NIH, provided him

28

with a pump oxygenator and the equipment necessary to perform open-heart surgery which he carried out in Cape Town. He acquired three years of salary and lab support to start his experiments. Before he left for Cape Town, he visited Dr. Lawler in the College of West Virginia and Dr. Shumway's laboratories in California to learn various experimental techniques and research in cardiac transplantation.

Dr. Shumway spent ten years in research working in basic areas to make heart transplant patients safe. He developed the preservation of the heart by surface cooling. He also designed a method whereby the heart could be biopsied through a hole to determine rejection. He also introduced Cyclosporin as an immunosuppression agent to allow suppression of the immune system to prevent rejection phenomenon. Dr. Shumway and Dr. Lawler also provided a means of arterial anastomosis where the heart atrial cap would be used for the anastomosis (put together) rather than seven anastamoses by different vessels that supply the heart. Thus, the two anastomoses procedure was developed and made heart transplantation much simpler to perform. Despite the fact that Dr. Lawler and Dr. Shumway had produced the research throughout their careers for cardiac transplantation, Dr. Christiaan Barnard upstaged them in December of 1967. Again, the Wangensteen influence prevailed. Many times, Dr. Wangensteen had two individuals working on the same problem or projects to provide competition. To date, there

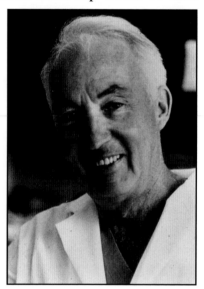

Dr. Shumway

have been 450 transplants carried out by Dr. Shumway who had an 80-90% one-year survival rate, and had a 60-70% five-year survival rate. Moreover, Christiaan Barnard was not operating fully at this time after his original transplant because of severe rheumatoid arthritis in his hands. His first assistant did a good deal of the heart transplant surgery in South Africa.

Through The Portals of Pigs and Manure

As an extension of Dr. Shumway's basic work, heart/lung transplants would also begin where a combination of organs were used for correction of difficult heart failure patients where lungs were involved and deficient in function.

Drs. C. Walt Lillehei, Christiaan Barnard and Denton Cooley all within a four year period had tried heart/lung transplants, however there were no survivors. In his laboratory, Dr. Shumway worked on heart/lung transplantation in primates and demonstrated feasibility of doing heart/lung transplants with the use of Cyclosporin as the immunosuppressive agent. Dr. Shumway then carried out the first living heart/lung transplant in 1981. Up to the present, half of them were still alive. So, the influence continues in Dr. Shumway's prototype working at the University of Minnesota under the Wangensteen program and then independently carried out research leading to these remarkable accomplishments.

Another interesting first in the area of open-heart surgery was the advent of the pacemaker. Dr. C. Walton Lillehei carried out open-heart surgery in the early 1950's. In repairing ventricular septal defects (a hole in the septum that divides the ventricles), and suturing around these defects, nerves responsible for the heartbeat were injured and created a heart rhythm defect called heart block. The heart would thus stop beating. Dr. Walt Lillehei expressed the need for some type of pacing device because of the injury to the nerves in the septum during the surgery of the ventricular septal defects, especially in cyanotic or "blue baby" children. Heart block occurred in several of these babies and they eventually died. At that time, Dr. Walt Lillehei used an AC power plug-in system, which was crude, but did result in heart stimulation. This lasted only a few hours, and in many instances burned the heart. In 1957 a power failure occurred at the University of Minnesota that resulted in a failure of his system, thus tremendous reduction in heart rate and shock to several patients who had this crude pacing system. They all had complicated cyanotic heart problems and had undergone open-heart corrective surgery. He contacted an engineer, Earl Bakken, who repaired pressure gauges and other monitoring equipment. He asked Earl Bakken if he could eliminate the direct AC current power cord, and Bakken came up with a car battery and a novel electrical system. This was the beginning of the pacemaker story. Earl Bakken took the electronics from a metronome (used normally for keeping a musical rhythm) and applied it to a stimulating electrode to produce heartbeats. The first system was worn outside on the patient's chest. This story will follow.

Thus the beginning of the open-heart era was born at the University of Minnesota with basic cardiac experimentation under the aegis of Dr. Maurice Visscher and with encouragement and funding by Dr. Wangensteen.

The success of the cardiac program also has to be attributed in part to the great cardiac pathologist, Dr. Jesse Edwards from the Mayo Clinic. His weekly meetings with the surgeons, pediatricians, and internists demonstrated the defects and mistakes made during surgery. His assessment of the problem was then responsible for correction of these complex congenital problems. Assessing these mistakes thus led to new advancements in the correction of the most complex heart problems. Dr. Wangensteen also encouraged him, and they became great friends. Dr. Edwards eventually started a heart bank for students and residents from all over the world to learn the basic problems before attempting complex cardiac surgery. Again, many firsts in cardiac surgery at the University of Minnesota began with this great combination of men dedicated to the field of open-heart surgery.

In the field of gastric physiology where Dr. Wangensteen was a giant, many of the students worked on the same problem. Dr. Varco and Dr. Code, working in physiology and in Dr. Wangensteen's lab, evaluated the use of histamine in beeswax as a chronic stimulator of hydrochloric acid, which the stomach parietal cells secrete. This gave an experimental preparation in the laboratory to evaluate various operative procedures for duodenal ulcers. This is one of the most important preparations created in Dr. Wangensteen's lab to study ulcer physiology.

Another of the most important contributions of Dr. Wangensteen was his experimental work in hypothermia. He was greatly influenced by the work of William Beaumont. In the 1850's, Dr. Beaumont was a pioneering American surgeon in the military outpost and his observations on Alexis St. Martin in 1853 ranked among the

Through The Portals of Pigs and Manure

finest contributions to gastric physiology. Alexis St. Martin had an open gastric fistula from a war wound (gastric juice spewed from the open wound). Dr. Beaumont's observation that the food stimulus elicited gastric secretion was important in understanding the concept in gastric physiology and the stimulus by vagus nerve (the cephalic phase). In another experimental design, a student of Dr. Wangensteen, Don Ferguson, in 1950 demonstrated that bathing of the cat's esophagus with warm gastric juice caused perforation regularly within two hours. If plain hydrochloric acid was used, there was only reddening. Thus, the catalytic effect of pepsin, an enzyme coupled with hydrochloric, was demonstrated as being important in the destruction of the mucosal (lining) tissue.

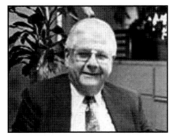

Dr. Ward Griffin

Dr. Ward Griffin and his associates demonstrated that when profusion juice was cooled, the mucosal damage by the warm gastric juice was eliminated. These observations by Dr. Wangensteen and his residents in the lab led to the use of gastric cooling for the prevention and treatment of gastric hemorrhage. These experiments also led to a clinical trial proving the effectiveness of cooling in reducing gastric ulcer hemorrhage. After the success of cooling, Dr. Wangensteen went one step further and reasoned that gastric freezing might improve the results of cooling. Although experimental work seemed to be helpful, human use of freezing was very controversial and resulted in perforations of stomach walls. These events led to the abandonment of the freezing concept.

An area that was quite obscure in the early 1960's was that of the central nervous influence on gastric secretion, a puzzle Dr. Wangensteen was intrigued with. I was greatly influenced by this concept and was also stimulated

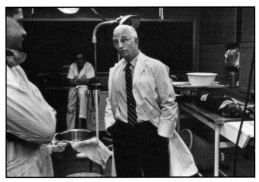

Dr. Ward Griffin and OHW

32

by Beaumont's observations. With the help of Dr. Donlin Long from the Department of Neurosurgery, who became head of neurosurgery at John Hopkins, we studied the influence of the central nervous system on gastric secretion. Dr. Wangensteen was very supportive of this pioneering work. Pavlov pouches (vagally innervated) were constructed in cats and electrodes were placed by stereotaxic technique in the brain area (hypothalamus) that controls parasympathetic (vagal) and sympathetic (adrenal) effect. We found that during anterior hypothalamic stimulation under low frequency, not only did gastric hydrochloric acid secretion increase, but this secretion decreased as the intensity of the stimulus increased (stress-like phenomenon). In addition, there was a decrease in blood flow with increased frequency. There was also alteration in protective stomach secretions by decrease in mucous factors (l. fucose sialic acid and hexosamine). The stress-type stimulation of the posterior hypothalamus produced a decrease in mucosal factors which protect the stomach from ulceration. This was in contrast to low frequency anterior hypothalamus stimulation (vagal) where there was a marked increase in gastric mucous factors. We thus suggested the pendular theory of stress ulcer. During a period of stress or posterior stimulation there was a marked decrease in acid secretion and gastric blood flow and when stressed is released, the anterior hypothalamus takes over and creates a vagal type effect with hyper secretion of hydrochloric and increase in gastric blood flow with

subsequent ulcer formation. Depending on the imbalance of factors and the severity of stress, the stomach was susceptible to ulcer formation. Ulcers were created in a cat by this intermittent type of vagal type stimulation. This was the subject of my own Ph.D. thesis and important in understanding stress ulcer formation. Dr. Wangensteen was intrigued and very supportive of this effort.

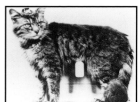

Cat with pouch and brain electrode

What about transplantation during the Wangensteen era? Dr. Richard Varco and the pediatric nephrologist team were interested in the origination of whole organ transplantation at the University of Minnesota. Drs. Richard Varco, Joe Aust, William Kelly and myself started kidney transplantation at the University of Minnesota in 1963. The first kidney transplantation was carried out on identical

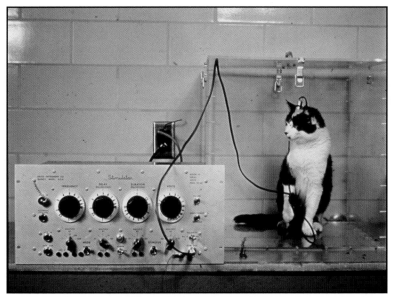

Stimulation apparatus stress ulcer lab experiment

twins, and no rejection was anticipated. I removed the kidney and Drs. Varco, Aust, and Kelly placed the transplanted kidney in the identical twin. Original work in pancreatic transplantation was carried out by Dr. Richard Lillehei who did the first whole pancreas transplant in 1966 after several years of experimental work supported by Dr. Wangensteen. Fourteen pancreatic transplants were carried out from 1966 to 1973.

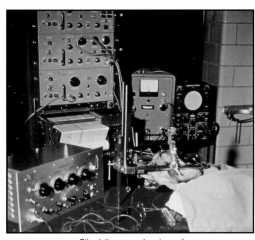

Stimulation apparatus stress ulcer

The transplant program flourished under the aegis of Dr. John Najarian who took over the Department of Surgery in 1967. Presently, forty years later, several thousand transplants of kidney, pancreas and liver have been carried out at the University of Minnesota. These

34

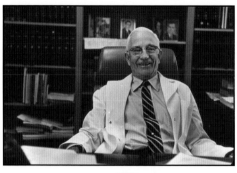

OHW

include several firsts by Dr. Najarian in diabetic kidney transplantation in children and in liver transplantation in children (see Najarian and Transplants). Dr. Wangensteen was very supportive of the original transplant work before his retirement. As you can see from the aforementioned projects, the Wangensteen influence continued. Many decisions were made when philosophies of the day were contrary.

Now, what did Dr. Wangensteen accomplish during his retirement? In an interview before he died, he fashioned himself as being a super annotated professor and wrote this to Dr. Evarts Graham who he teamed up with to start the surgical forum. After retirement, he was able to relax, travel, and visit historical European surgical schools. He visited many of his former students in their departmental duties. When he returned in 1967, Dr. Wangensteen also helped provide the University with funds for a history of medicine professorship. Moreover, he helped to provide the funds and much of the stimulus for the growth of one of the finest History of Medicine Departments and libraries in the country.

Through The Portals of Pigs and Manure

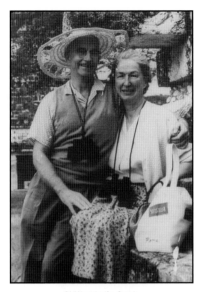

OHW and wife, Sarah

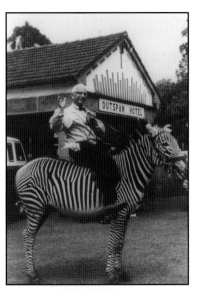

OHW on vacation

He and his wife Sarah, one of the most knowledgable medical editors, completed a major book on the history of surgery entitled, "The Rise of Surgery from an Empiric Craft to a Scientific Discipline." What could be a more fitting title to describe Dr. Wangensteen's monumental contributions in surgery? Just before his death in January of 1981, I asked him, if given another chance, would he repeat his career. He said, "Yes, by all means. But only if I could have my devoted wife, Sarah with me." He said he felt academic life was the most challenging arena in which to be given the privilege to work. Finally in Dr. Wangensteen's own

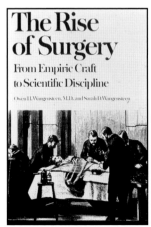

The Rise of Surgery
From Empiric Craft
to Scientific Discipline

Owen H. Wangensteen, M.D. and Sarah D. Wangensteen

Book by OHW and his wife, Sarah

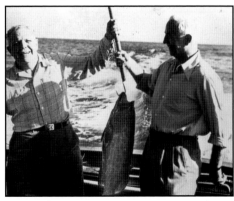

OHW enjoying a fishing trip with Dr. Graham

words, "May we by example and precept awaken in each of you an eagerness to excel in all aspects of your accepted trust. May all of us come to know the abundant rewards of shared opportunity, the finest of paymasters. May each of us through prudent and thrifty living come to know the satisfaction and contentment of sharing our bounty in good causes and especially with institutions that created for us the presence of opportunity to spend our lives in the service of our fellow men and women." Dr. Wangensteen's influence and stimulus will resound in the years to come and will stimulate many minds in basic surgical disciplines.

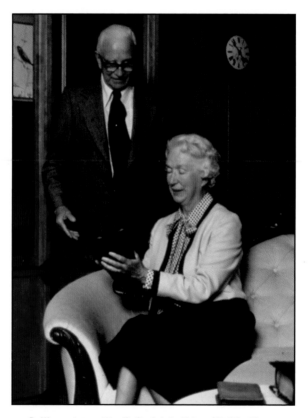

Dr. Wangensteen and his wife, Sarah, in the History of Medicine Library

Chapter 2

Personal Observations by Dr. Wangensteen's Staff Assistant, Mildred Jones

My ten years of observing Dr. Wangensteen in his capacity as teacher, researcher, and administrator have brought me to three outstanding explanations for his success: (1) his personal work habits and the value he placed on time; an economy which enables him to achieve the maximum from any given 24 hours, (2) his Spartan-like thrift which, when imposed rigidly on everyone from himself to the last office clerk and laboratory aid, enabled him to amass extra funds for the important research projects going on in his laboratories during those years, and (3) his almost unfailing ability to assess character and intelligence, a gift which enabled him to surround himself with young doctors and scientists of the caliber necessary to accept the challenge of a demanding research lab.

Dr. Wangensteen regarded time as a valuable commodity and never tolerated a slackening of the almost inhuman pace he set for himself and his staff – including secretaries. I remember him coming up from the operating room or the laboratories and passing through our office like a bolt of lightning, calling out to the receptionist as he headed for his own inner office to get Dr. So & So on the phone, have his resident come up in an hour, look up someone's credentials in the A.M.A. directory, pull the file on the new resident application, etc. His orders usually lasted until he entered his private office and shut the door, leaving the receptionist frantically trying to write everything down. It was important to hear him right the first time! Dr. Wangensteen did not tolerate being asked to repeat an order. Indeed, if the secretary had summoned the courage to follow him into his office to clarify something, she would have found him already engrossed in the his next problem, and the red "do not disturb" light blazing from the intercom on his desk. One observant resident once remarked that Dr. Wangensteen had only to enter the office and "all hell broke loose." It could indeed, and often did, especially when he

38

was in the process of putting together the necessary paper work for application for research funds and training grants or justifying their continued funding.

It is well known that Dr. Wangensteen worked on research problems for his laboratory during the wee hours at his home and often came to work filled with ideas for new projects. Some of his most startling and dramatic experiments began in this way (the cooling and freezing treatment for ulcers, for example). The administrative work involved in running a department was treated in the same manner, particularly in regard to research papers, progress reports, and grant proposals. This type of work usually went into his Scotch plaid handbag (no fancy briefcase) to be dealt with during the predawn hours at home.

Dr. Wangensteen did all of his own writing and editing during these years as surgeon, researcher, and administrator of department affairs. The era of the Editorial Assistant had not yet arrived. He always came into the office with pages and pages of yellow paper scribbled in his very difficult, cramped handwriting, and asked for a typed copy as soon as possible – that usually meant within an hour. The Office Supervisor often had to divide the yellow sheets among the secretaries to have it typed in OHW rough style (6 spaces between lines) and have it done soon enough to suit Dr. Wangensteen. No one went to break, lunch, or even "down the hall" to the washroom until Dr. Wangensteen's paper was done. It might be of interest to note here that Dr. Wangensteen's spelling and choice of words were faultless. We never had to double-check or rearrange his words to make smoother sentences. He did cling to the use of some archaic words (the word "anent" for instance) but new typists soon became familiar with them. He also clung to an almost outmoded use of punctuation (e.g., he always put a comma after the word "that"). He was very rigid as far as punctuation was concerned and always insisted the typist copy his work exactly as he indicated. It was his tedious scribbled handwriting that slowed us down; we often found it necessary to have an experienced secretary work with newcomers and "translate" for them.

Through The Portals of Pigs and Manure

Dr. Wangensteen's constant fight with time – to make it yield the maximum in any given period – made itself felt throughout the office and often left tired and exhausted employees in his wake, for like most brilliant men, he vastly underestimated the average rate of production. He was intolerant of slower intellect, the shy, and the inarticulate. For this reason we tried to surround him with secretaries who could respond quickly and recall with reasonable accuracy. The Office Supervisor, a controversial figure, served for many years as liaison between Dr. Wangensteen, the rest of the staff, his personal secretary, and the receptionist, another controversial figure but one who had a quick mind and aggressive nature. Even though we felt the brunt of his ambitious drive, I heard very little griping among the secretaries, even at times when we were most driven. We realized he held himself to the same rigid rules he imposed on everyone else, and somehow this made it easier to meet his demands.

Dr. Wangensteen's passion for economy and thrift did not stop with his use of time. He abhorred waste of funds and materials and permitted no frills or unnecessary items in any of the offices. His own office was uncarpeted and equipped with good but strictly utilitarian furniture. This was characteristic of him during those days, for the aesthetic always seemed to be sacrificed in Dr. Wangensteen's scheme of things. I have never heard of him attending a concert, theatre, or art show, or associated in any way with other than medical events. His tremendous drive was always trained in one direction, which may be one reason for his success. Those of us who worked in the "main" office will remember how he held the reins on office equipment. The need for new typewriters, or office furniture, had to be well demonstrated before we could expect approval for replacements like the verifax machine, the forerunner of modern duplicating machines, and portable tape dictating machines for his own use. Only when he was persuaded that these items would "save time" did he permit them to be purchased. Convenience machines like our power files of today, electric stapling machines, electric pencil sharpeners and can openers would certainly have been denied. He insisted office supplies be conserved, however allowed lavish use of yellow paper (because it was cheap, he said) and always used it himself for rough copies, and first drafts. Even "Department of Surgery" notepaper was used with discrimination; Dr. Wangensteen usually scribbled his interoffice notes on little scraps of paper. When he received a book one day from one of our Professors with certain pages marked for his attention with "Dept. of Surgery" printed notepaper, he called a secretary in, showed her the book and asked her to tell the professor not to use good department notepaper for bookmarks, He used scraps of yellow paper and would advise others to do the same.

Dr. Wangensteen disciplined his personal life in the same manner. His car was small, in keeping with the size of his family, his modest River Road home, his habits conservative. He seemed to deplore ostentation, the obvious display of wealth, and what he considered a waste of money. This was clearly demonstrated when he and Mrs. Wangensteen accepted an invitation to dinner at the home of his Office Supervisor, a woman of considerable private wealth. He was aghast at the wealthy décor of her beautiful home, and was absolutely astounded at a display of her expensive hobby – a collection of rare dolls from all over the world. Compared to his own hobby – the collection of rare medical books that redeemed themselves by their historical value, collecting dolls seemed to be an extremely unrewarding and nonproductive pastime. A more objective appraisal would have had to admit the dolls might have had a historical interest also, evident in their costumes, headdress, and coiffures, etc., representing one period or another. But Dr. Wangensteen was not objective, he was very frank in his disapproval of the hobby, and it seemed to disturb his evening. He must have worried about it during the night, for the next morning he strode into the office and told the Supervisor at least she could sell those "damn dolls" if she ever needed money. Such "irresponsible" use of money was incomprehensible to him and he preferred to regard it as a business investment.

Dr. Wangensteen's schemes for bringing money into the department for teaching and research would have done credit to master fundraisers. His Annual Research Luncheons, to which the financial giants of the Twin Cities were invited and made acquainted with the work going on in the labs always brought renewed funds to keep the work going. The laboratory projects, fifteen or twenty of them usually, were explained to this distinguished audience in lay terms by the brilliant young doctors involved in them. They addressed the audience in five minute speeches during the luncheon and afterwards stood near exhibits of their projects designed to help the unsophisticated grasp some idea of the fascination and mystery in a research lab. Scrubbed, brushed, and shining, these young resident doctors from the laboratories used to make themselves available, attentive and generally charming to the wealthy visitors, much to Dr. Wangensteen's delight. The annual luncheons created a spirit of goodwill among the philanthropists of Minneapolis and St. Paul, and the experimental labs of the Surgery Deptartment reaped financial benefits.

Another source of income stemmed from Dr. Wangensteen's practice of channeling donations from grateful and wealthy patients or their families and friends directly into funds for research. Also funds were used for travel to scientific meetings for his residents, or to cover other lab expenditures not provided for in federal monies. His zeal in garnering support along with his meticulous attention to expenditures assured the continuation of his projects. Indeed, his careful administration of research grants, training grants, and volunteer funds enabled him to turn over a financially sound department to his successor Dr. Najarian, in 1967.

Dr. Wangensteen's accomplishments have been phenomenal, but he could not have done it alone. He needed extensions of himself in his labs and operating rooms – extensions he fashioned in the superior brains and talented hands of the men he chose from his roster of surgery residents. For many years Dr. Wangensteen personally interviewed resident applications and only the most promising candidates received his approval for the intensive seven year ordeal called "residency." His keen eye summed up a man's character quickly and accurately and enabled him to choose only the most brilliant for his resident staff, and later only the sharpest of these to train in his own lab under his personal direction. However, now and then he accepted a candidate simply because he felt the young man had something special to offer. The story has often been told of how a young man applied for a residency and received it in spite of the fact that he was obviously not residential material in any way. He had already failed in an effort to work in a partnership arrangement with several other doctors in a small town, and the grades on his transcript from Medical School were barely mediocre, but Dr. Wangensteen sensed something about the intense, almost ascetic young man, and accepted him for residency. Instead of admitting him normally in graduate school, Dr. Wangensteen hired him as a deaner in the lab. His persuasive letter on behalf of the young applicant to the Dean to let him in the surgery program was considered a classic. Everyone knows the ending – this particular resident, Dr. Richard Dewall, worked in Drs. Wangensteen and Lillehei's labs and eventually invented the bubble pump oxygenator which made open heart surgery possible.

Dr. Wangensteen's keen insight into character also enabled him to handle the members of his faculty staff and maintain a tight control of the direction in which the department moved in spite of internal politics. Those of us who worked in his "main" offices often watched as some prominent staff member emerged from his private office red-faced and obviously bested in an eyeball-to-eyeball confrontation with the Chief. From our vantage point we noted other things. We knew if any of his staff had special training or skills, he made use of them to further his work – e.g., if a staff member knew several languages, such as Dr. Aldo Castaneda, Dr. Wangensteen made use of that knowledge by sending him books and articles to be read and summarized and translated in English for him. For many years he was one of the editors of the journal, Surgery and obligated to review manuscripts submitted for publication. The staff man known to be involved in the area of investigation concerned in the manuscript was usually asked to review and evaluate the paper with a recommendation for acceptance or rejection. We knew he made use of certain undesirable characteristics of at least one employee in the department. His receptionist of many years, was generally known to be extremely aggressive and rude, and never hesitated to be insulting if she felt so disposed. To her he sometimes turned over problems like the lazy resident – bullying him into keeping to the departmental schedules, turning in reports, showing up at lectures, and conferences – thus minor violations of discipline beneath the dignity of Chief to notice and reprimand in single instances but which interfered with the smooth, on-going flow of departmental function. At a word or two from Dr. Wangensteen, the receptionist began to "take care of the problem," insulting, belittling, embarrassing, and generally hounding him until the poor recalcitrant resident fell in line and stayed there in order to avoid the hassle. Thus, Dr. Wangensteen affected desired ends by using this particular employee's most objectionable traits. Unfortunately, she also insulted and embarrassed others, but Dr. Wangensteen turned deaf ears to all complaints. This is one illustration of the fact he placed the department and its functions, its development, and its welfare, before the comfort of employees and staff – indeed, before his own comfort. This is consistent with other facets of his long administration, and perhaps one secret of his tremendous success.

Chapter 3

Dr. Lester Dragstedt Interview
Dr. Wangensteen's Contributions in Intestinal Obstruction, Ulcer Physiology, Cancer, and his Fundamental Approach to Resident Training

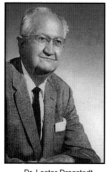

Dr. Lester Dragstedt

Dr. Lester Dragstedt, who was a professor and the head of surgery at the University of Chicago and an excellent gastrointestinal surgeon and gastric physiologist was a close friend of Dr. Wangensteen. In an interview at Dr. Wangensteen's home, I asked Dr. Dragstedt what he felt Dr. Wangensteen's greatest contribution was, clinically. Without hesitation, he felt Dr. Wangensteen's introduction of a method to decompress the stomach after abdominal operations was his greatest clinical achievement. This method produced physiologic significance and Dr. Dragstedt also adopted the innovation in his practice. He would observe immediate relief of pain and commented in his patients, the suction system prevented postoperative ileus (continuous dilated bowel). He used it until patients recovered bowel activity. He felt this was Dr. Wangensteen's greatest contribution to American surgery. It is now used worldwide.

For centuries, it was a mystery on how to treat patients with distension of the abdomen by mechanical causes such as adhesions, tumors, dilatation of the bowel from infection, stress, or postoperative bowel paralysis. This problem stimulated Dr. Wangensteen at an early age while a resident in surgery awaiting his future appointment as an instructor in surgery. He wanted to figure out a method of bowel decompression or relief of gaseous collections in the bowel from any of the above causes. He developed a gastric siphonage system with a tube inserted into the stomach through the nose. This experimental design was the first great contribution he developed based on pathophysiologic observation. His fame spread quickly in the University and surgical world as early as the 1930's. He first published his work in an obscure Wisconsin medical publication, having been turned down by the major surgical journals of the time. This apparatus was eventually used by clinics and hospitals all over the United States and world and it was used preoperatively to prevent aspiration of obstructed intestinal content. It was used postoperatively in major abdominal surgery to prevent so called intestinal ileus (paralyzed gut with accumulation of gas). This discovery alone was responsible for saving thousands of lives and preventing the numerous complications of intestinal obstruction of all kinds.

Continuing in the intestinal obstruction problem, Wangensteen was perplexed with the inability to decompress the mechanically obstructed or paralyzed small bowel prior to surgery. At surgery, once the abdomen was opened, the surgeon was greeted with enormously distended bowel filled with gas and secretions. I was in the lab at the time, and received the assignment from Dr. Wangensteen to evaluate the problem, which meant, "do something about it." A Miller-Abbott rubber tube had been used with little success. It was flimsy and if no activity in the bowel was present, the tube could not be advanced prior to surgical intervention. There was a need for decompression of gas and fluid to allow the operator a clear field to carry out his or her exploration.

The problem was that in a rubber tube, a wire could not be introduced or extracted because of friction in the tube wall. I designed a coil spring (wire) plastic tube (Leonard long tube) with a bulbous tip and a balloon to which a piano wire could be placed and extracted, as metal on metal provided very little friction and the wire had inherent flexibility. Dr. Wangensteen was emphatic regarding immediate clinical use. By the 1960's, the device was tested on several patients with immediate success. The first publication introducing this technique in surgical patients was in 1961. Dr. Richard Edlich used this tube for non-operative decompression in a series of patients in 1962 and Dr. Robert Goodale in 1967 was able to place the tube

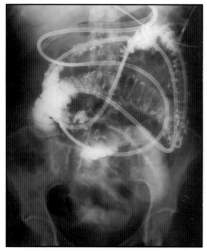
Leonard long coiled spring tube

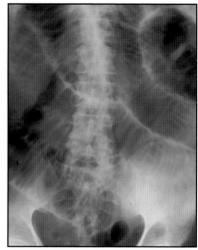
X-ray of obstructed abdomen

endoscopically in the duodenum so preoperative decompression could be carried out. Constant encouragement by Dr. Wangensteen was responsible for the successful use of this device for intestinal obstruction, mechanical or ileus (paralyzed bowel full of gas). Dr. Dragstedt praised this technique.

Another area where Dr. Wangensteen excelled was querying the unknown in the origin of appendicitis. Historically, many theories in this area had been proposed. Dr. Wangensteen felt the obstruction of the appendix was by facalith (firm round secretion residing in the appendix). He suggested a series of experiments to test his theory. He and one of his first residents, Dr. Clarence Dennis proved his theory by ligating the appendix in animals (apes) and measuring the appendicle pressures necessary to perforate the organ. In the obstructed appendix, it took two times the systolic pressure, and perforation occurred within two hours. These pressures shut off the blood supply of the appendicle wall, which led to deterioration and finally perforation. Again, Dr. Wangensteen's approach of applying experimental means to solving an old theoretic suggestion brought credence to the medical arena. Thus, Dr. Wangensteen became a student in many areas of intestinal obstruction. His work and his book on intestinal obstruction is a classic. Dr. Dragstedt brought up this historical solution of an ancient problem.

Through The Portals of Pigs and Manure

In my interview with Dr. Dragstedt, I asked what other major influences Dr. Wangensteen and his students had on American surgery during his tenure. Dr. Dragstedt felt Drs. Code and Varco's experimental work in the 1940's, using pellets of histamine and beeswax to stimulate gastric hydrochloric acid was a superb contribution to gastric physiology and an understanding of the ulcer problem. Their experiments, using histamine and beeswax as the stimulating agent, confirmed a marked increase in gastric hydrochloric acid secretion by their method. Dragstedt used this technique experimentally to confirm the effect of vagotomy as an operation to decrease duodenal ulcer formation. Clinically, night secretion in these highly stressed ulcer patients was reduced by vagotomy. Dragstedt's first operative vagotomy in an ulcer patient was carried out in 1943 and was indeed successful. Wangensteen however, preferred gastrectomy (stomach resection) as treatment for ulcers, predicting vagotomy alone was not sufficient treatment. This was verified in a randomized series experimentally and clinically.

Dr. Wangensteen designed several types of gastric operations using the histamine and beeswax experimentally to prove the efficiency of these operations. He and Dr. Dragstedt had many discussions on which method was the best treatment. Dr. Wangensteen's fundamental experimental approach impressed Dr. Dragstedt and the American College professors. Dr. Dragstedt was also impressed with Dr. Wangensteen's principles in the treatment of cancer in those early pre-radiation and chemotherapy years, namely wide resection of disease and the inclusion of radical resection of lymph nodes in the area of the cancer. He also mentioned Dr. Wangensteen's approach to cancer after the initial operation, the so-called second look procedure, where six months after initial resection of cancer, patients were re-explored and a thorough search was undertaken for any gross residual cancer. These were long and tedious procedures, some lasting twelve hours. Today, we have CT scans, PET scans, MRI's, and radioactive scans that in most instances take the place of the second look approach.

After observing Dr. Wangensteen's surgery department training progress with residents spending two to three years in experimental surgery and the testing of new ideas, Dr. Dragstedt pressed for this new teaching and development of surgeons approach at the American College of Surgeons. He and Dr. Evarts Graham, President of the American College of Surgeons, reiterated the great value of the surgical forum at the college meetings. This discipline allowed young people to present their research and be criticized by the "surgical greats of the time." Heretofore, the meetings were devoted to dissertations by the older members of the society and the younger members were supposed to listen and learn. These latter sessions were mostly clinical, not research based. Thus, the forum was a great advance in the surgical discipline where fledgling fellows were exposed to fundamental problem solving. As Dr. Wangensteen suggested, it changed surgery from an empirical craft to a scientific discipline, out of which came the Minnesota origin of open-heart surgery, the pacemaker, and the pump oxygenator, as examples. Dragstedt described Wangensteen as the most colorful figure in American surgery.

Chapter 4

The Ulcer Story

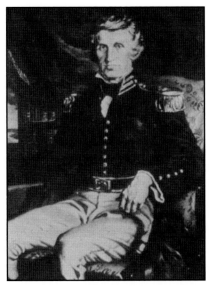
Dr. William Beaumont

Early in Dr. Owen H. Wangensteen's career, he was fascinated with the problem of a duodenal ulcer. His insatiable desire to probe history and kindle scientific based treatments of the problem led him to probe the history of Dr. William Beaumont, a civil war surgeon and Alexis St. Martin, a Native American who had a gastric fistula (stomach opening to the outside) caused by a battle wound. He visioned an approach using Pavlov pouches (vagal type) as an extension of this history to study the ulcer problem.

He also was intrigued by Dr. John Hunter who was one of the great historical originators of probing the pathophysiology of disease process by observation and experimentation. He also recounted the work of Pavlov, the father of brain or central nervous stimulation by the vagal nerve, as a possible approach to ulcer disease. Dr. Beaumont observed as follows. As Alexis St. Martin was exposed to food, his gastric fistula secreted much more juice. He concluded there was indeed a cause and effect. He reasoned the brain, through a stimulation process, eventually turned out to be the vagal or parasympathetic effect on gastric secretions (mainly hydrochloric acid). This story and observation led to a number of experiments by Dr. Owen H. Wangensteen and another great gastric physiologist, Dr. Lester Dragstedt. It also became the basis of several experiments in the laboratory to evaluate the origin of gastric secretion and the effect of the vagus nerve in altering secretion. These observations and experiments led to an understanding of the cause of the duodenal ulcer, and eventual treatment approaches.

The Story of the Minnesota Influence on American Surgery

Dr. Wangensteen stimulated Dr. Richard Varco who at that time was a young resident scientist, to study these phenomena in the laboratory in the late 1940's. In the physiology lab, Dr. Varco and Dr. Code used histamine and beeswax in experiments to produce a duodenal ulcer. Histamine stimulated the parietal cells (hydrochloric acid producing cells in the stomach). Beeswax allowed a chronic or continuous stimulating phase. Pellets were created to be used in a variety of experimental procedures to produce the ulcer diathesis. Thus, this became an important model to evaluate and to treat the duodenal ulcer.

Dr. Wangensteen then used this preparation to design several operative gastric procedures to cure the duodenal ulcer. This included the 75% gastric resection where the majority of parietal cells were resected. Meanwhile, Dr. Wangensteen experimented on the cutting of the vagal nerve (the nerve from the stomach) which stimulated the parietal or hydrochloric secreting cells. He also found that the vagus nerve stimulated stomach contraction and when cut, caused partial obstruction to the outlet of the stomach. Thus, he created a less invasive procedure – vagotomy (cutting of the vagus nerve) and pyloroplasty (opening of the distal part of the stomach) which became one of the standard operative procedures for ulcer disease. At Chicago University, Dr. Dragstedt also used this model to study the effects of vagotomy.

In my own lab with the encouragement of Dr. Wangensteen, we studied the brain (or central nervous system) effect on stress ulcer by putting probes in the hypothalamus, which is the central brain control center of the vagus nerve that also controls the area for stress or sympathetic effect on stomach secretion. When stimulated, this stress area essentially stops secretion. By stereotaxis, using a device to place probes in the hypothalamus (the base of the brain control center),

GASTRIC PHYSIOLOGY

CNS INFLUENCE IN GASTRIC SECRETION

1. ANT. HYPOTHALAMUS
   (VAGAL AREA)
   a) ↑ HCL SECRETION
   b) ↓ BLOOD FLOW AS
      INC. FREQUENCY
2. POST HYPOTHALAMUS
   a) ↓ HCL SECRETION

PENDULAR THEORY

STRESS ULCER

Gastric Physiology Experiment

51

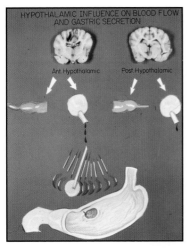

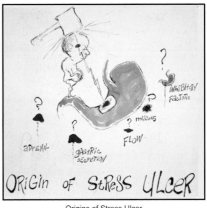

Origins of Stress Ulcer

Hypothalamic Influence on Blood Flow
and Gastric Secretion

Dr. Donlin Long, a neurosurgery resident, who eventually became head of neurosurgery at John Hopkins University, worked with me. I created Pavlov pouches (like that of Alexis St. Martin's fistula) which were vagally innervated. We found that low frequency stimulation in the anterior hypothalamus of the brain created marked gastric secretion increase. By high frequency stimulation of the anterior, vagal or parasympathetic area of the hypothalamus, secretion was shut off. Posteriorly, hypothalamic stimulation itself stopped secretion (stress area). Then, if one waited after high frequency stimulation was stopped, and observed the pouch secretions, a rebound effect occurred with a marked increase in acid secretion. We subsequently observed the formation of many small ulcers. We called this phenomenon the pendular pattern of gastric secretion and the basis of stress ulcer. We also resected the antrum in these stimulation experiments. This distal part of the stomach secreted gastrin, which was the hormonal stimulus to gastric secretion, and by resection we were able to prevent ulcer formation. These basic ulcer experiments as previously stated, became the basis of my Ph.D.. thesis emanating from original encouragement and suggestions from Dr. Wangensteen. Vagotomy and antrectomy were eventually used as one of the surgical treatments for ulcer disease. The experimental designs gave basis for treatment. Other gastric physiologists had already studied the hormone phase (gastrin) of stomach secretion. Wangensteen always gave credit to his pupils and encouraged their basic physiologic probing for the basis of understanding and treating disease.

Another problem with ulcer formation was bleeding. Dr. Wangensteen again was fascinated by the historical experiments of Dr. John Hunter on cooling the stomach and its effect on secretion. He considered an experimental approach to see the effect of cooling on the formation of ulcer and bleeding. Dr. Peter Salmon, and Dr. Ward Griffin, residents in Dr. Wangensteen's lab and others began by observing that

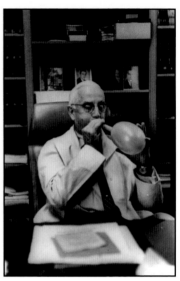

Dr. Wangensteen and cooling balloon

cooling also decreased the destructive acid effect on the distal part of the esophagus. He reasoned that cooling depressed gastric secretion. A gastric balloon was developed and a cooling machine pumped cool fluid into the balloon. Dr. Wangensteen immediately introduced the concept clinically. Gastric bleeding was depressed or halted. A large clinical series by Dr. Robert Goodale produced excellent results in the control of gastric bleeding for ulcer disease. This is yet another concept that was based on the Wangensteen method of using history to query the unknown.

Following the cooling experiments and the successful clinical approach, Wangensteen questioned that if cooling was successful, what would be the effect of gastric freezing? Although experiments in the laboratory by Dr. Bernstein and Dr. Edwards seemed encouraging, Wangensteen was determined early to clinically apply the process. Unfortunately this concept proved disastrous, with a number of gastric or stomach perforations ensuing. A Mayo clinical series and other freezing series served to stop this treatment.

This survey of ulcer-based experiments was typical on the Wangensteen approach to basic problems and led to many successful clinical treatments. This is another example of the Minnesota influence on American surgery.

Chapter 5
The Cancer Detection Center

Dr. Wangensteen became disenchanted after many gross long operations for cancer (before the advent of chemotherapy) that late diagnosis was present in most of these cases. However, he was impressed by the fact that when experienced personnel found early breast lesions in women who were examined at regular intervals, they had five-year survival rates close to 90%. Eventually, mammograms were able to pick up lesions before they could be felt. The yearly application of the cervical papanicolaou smear had improved the cervical cancer survival rate in women. Also, the application of routine rectal and distal large bowel endoscopy had reduced mortality significantly. The use of routine air contrast colon exams eventually had helped in decreasing colon cancer mortality.

Despite these facts, Dr. Wangensteen felt the need for a cancer detection center where routine interval exams in the above areas of breast, cervical, and colon would bring marked improvement to the mortality of this dreadful disease. By the time palpable or systemic disease is found in clinic practice, the lesions have been present at least two years or more with spread most likely present. Thus, he felt the survival rate would be reduced significantly by examinations at regular intervals.

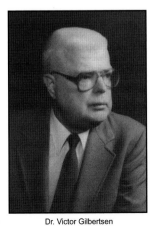
Dr. Victor Gilbertsen

Dr. Wangensteen tried to establish a cancer detection clinic as early as World War Two. Unfortunately, for monetary reasons the faculty disapproved and it was three years before this cancer detection center became a reality. The American Cancer Society did not have funds available to support the idea and it took three decades to get national funding for the project. Dr. Victor Gilbertsen was in charge. Routine colorectal, breast and cervical exams were

54

studied. Stools were processed for blood. He studied 475 patients. 10% of patients had recurrent blood in stools. Almost all patients had early cancer of the mucosal variety without obvious spread. The follow-up in all these patients with early lesions demonstrated the importance of early detection with above 90% survival. How important it would be to establish these detection centers today.

In Japan, early detection of gastric or stomach cancers in their gastroenterology clinics decreased mortality. Today, gastroscopy should be able to detect early lesions in the stomach and routine colorectal endoscopy should find early colon lesions.

The Wangensteen concept of cancer detection centers should be adopted with the advent of modern endoscopy and radiologic advances. This should not be limited to one area of the body but be combined in a cancer detection comprehensive clinic. It is disappointing that clinics such as these are not established throughout the country. The cost of early detection is a fraction of the cost for chemotherapy, radiation therapy, aggressive surgery, and loss of quality of life.

Chapter 6
The Heart Story

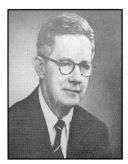

Dr. Alfred Blalock

The first closed heart procedure was carried out by Dr. Robert Gross in 1938. This was a closure of the ductus arteriosis (a congenital union of the subclavian artery to the pulmonary artery) which could cause early heart failure. This was followed by a closed heart procedure by Dr. Alfred Blalock in 1944, where in "blue babies" (tetralogy of Fallot) he developed a procedure suturing the subclavian artery to the pulmonary artery. This procedure brought oxygenated blood to the lungs. These men therefore expanded the scope of early heart surgery by these closed heart procedures with very sick babies and children. Surgeons were eager to perform open-heart surgery to correct these complex congenital heart problems where the heart needed oxygenated blood to pump to the brain and other vital organs. Thus, some type of artificial oxygenation was needed to give time for the surgeon to correct the defects by opening the heart. The closed heart procedures were only temporary fixes.

At Jefferson Medical College of Philadelphia, one of the first attempts to correct this problem was by Dr. John Gibbon. He innovated a heart/lung machine (oxygenator) and by 1947 was able to support animals in the laboratory using this heart/lung bypass device, but only for a few minutes. At the same time, Dr. Clarence Dennis at the University of Minnesota had built a heart/lung machine which was tested in the lab from the encouragement of Dr. Wangensteen. He used the device on a six year old with an atrial septal defect (upper heart defect). At the time, lab procedures were encouraged to go clinical without national approval by the FDA. The six year old patient developed pulmonary edema and heart failure, most likely from high pulmonary (lung) pressure and died. Dr. Gibbon experienced the same problem on a number of patients he attempted open-heart surgery. So, no means of bypassing the heart with these heart/lung devices were yet successful to give adequate operative time to correct the severe congenital heart defects.

56

In 1950, Dr. Bigelow in Toronto, used hypothermia (lowering of blood temperature) in dogs to extend the time one could use to operate on complex defects and save the brain. However, that method only gave a few minutes time for surgery in the heart. The first successful open heart surgery in the world was performed at the University of Minnesota on September 21, 1952. This was accomplished by Drs. Richard Varco, John Lewis, and Monseur Taufic on an interatrial septal defect in a five year old girl under hypothermia (cooling the body). Prior to this case, Dr. Lewis, like Dr. Bigelow, had performed numerous experiments on dogs in the lab using hypothermia. Dr. F. John Lewis et.al. performed eleven open hearts using this technique which resulted in two deaths. Dr. Wangensteen was very supportive of this work and encouraged new horizons of research to extend the time for these procedures.

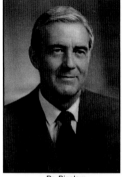

Dr. Bigelow

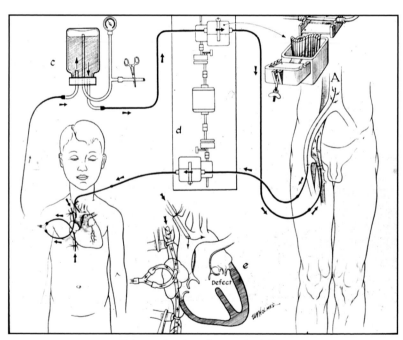

Scheme drawing of cross circulation

Through The Portals of Pigs and Manure

Although hypothermia was an efficent way to decrease brain damage during these short periods of blood stasis (no perfusion during the procedure) as stated above, a different approach was necessary to give more operative time. More complex defects required some type of heart/lung bypass. Dr. Maurice Visscher, head of cardiac physiology at the University of Minnesota, taught and inspired teams that led to the first successful complex open heart surgeries at the University of Minnesota.

Drs. C. Walt Lillehei, Dr. Morley Cohen, and Herbert Warden experimented with a unique approach to gain time for surgical correction of more complex defects. At first Dr. Norm Crisp tried using single lung lobes as a means of bypass for perfusion of the body, but

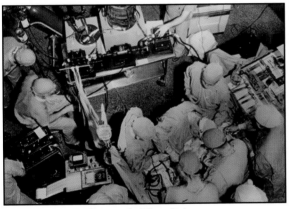

First cross circulation patient

failed to gain time. The breakthrough came when Drs. Warden, Cohen and Lillehei, under the direction of Dr. Maurice Visscher, used cross circulation where a donor animal provided oxygenated blood to the recipient with the heart defect.

A special pump provided the correct volume of blood between the two animals. Very few dogs died in contrast to the heart/lung pumps of Gibbon and Dennis. The donor dog needed to be five times the weight of the recipient for adequate perfusion (blood supply to the body). After success in the laboratory to gain time for fixing of complex defects, Dr. Lillehei called Dr. Wangensteen to report this success and asked for permission to try the technique on a sick one year old boy with a "blue baby" defect. Dr. Wangensteen was encouraging and sent a note to Lillehei. "By all means Walt, go ahead. Good luck." He demonstrated his undying faith in his young innovative residents and staff. You can imagine this aggressive approach today would be greatly inhibited by delay in FDA approval, and delay in approval by several committees necessary to gain permission. Months might have passed.

This whole approach was experimental based on the physiologic principle taught by Dr. Maurice Visscher, that minimal blood flow through the pulmonary vein in the heart during bypass was enough to prevent organ failure and brain damage during the bypass procedure. This approach of experimentally using a dog and subsequently a human as the heart/lung bypass gained precious time for the correction of complex cardiac defects.

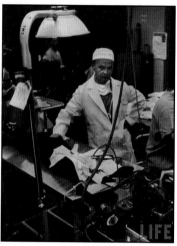

C. Walt Lillehei in lab - cross circulation experiment

The first human (a one year old boy) was operated on in March of 1954. The operation was successful, but he died of pneumonia eleven days after bypass surgery. Dr. Lillehei's team was encouraged by the successful operation, and used this technique on eight patients with complex defects of the ventricle and one blue baby with tetrology of Fallot. Even though all of these patients were in poor condition, only two died. This was a remarkable beginning to the open-heart surgery era. Dr. Wangensteen was delighted and showed his usual support of his young staff and their research based entrance to clinical fields yet to be conquered. Parents were used as donors and needed to be five times the recipient's weight to give enough perfusion to prevent brain and organ failure. A heart/lung machine was still needed because of the risk in humans for donor perfusion.

Dr. Richard Dewall, a young physician in general practice in Anoka, was interested in coming to the Wangensteen program. He applied to the graduate school but was turned down by Dr. Blegen, head of the University graduate education program. He had graduated in the lower half of his class. At the time, one needed to be in the upper 25% of the class for entrance into graduate school. All of the prior heart team was in the graduate program working on their Ph.D. degrees under Drs.Wangensteen and Visscher.

Through The Portals of Pigs and Manure

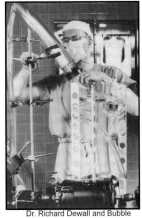

Dr. Richard Dewall and Bubble Oxygenator

Dr. Dewall came to Dr. Wangensteen with his idea of a bubble oxygenator. Impressed with his idea, Wangensteen hired Dr. Dewall as a deaner in the lab (animal attendant). Dr. Wangensteen always found creative ways to support his students with innovative approaches. Dr. Dewall went to the lab under the direction of Dr. Lillehei and Dr. Visscher and devised the bubble oxygenator, a big breakthrough for open-heart surgery. With laboratory support under Wangensteen and direction from Dr. Lillehei, experiments progressed. The principle of oxygen bubbles passing through blood into a coiled plastic device with silicone to de-bubble the blood before it was passed to the patient became the principle for a state of the art oxygenator.

The first patients were perfused in May of 1955. This opened a whole new future for open-heart surgery. For the first time, the oxygenator allowed the time necessary to repair complex congenital defects as well as repair or replacement of heart valves and later carry out coronary artery repairs. No human was needed, therefore, to be the bypass donor.

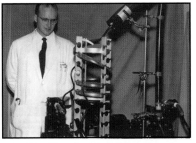

Dr. Richard Dewall and the Bubble Oxygenerator

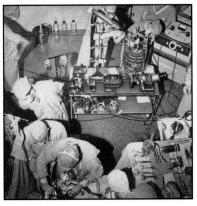

First bubble oxygenator operation

The program at the University was underway for the training of surgeons from around the country and the world. All of these techniques were lab based under the encouragement and support of Dr. Wangensteen. During a two to three year interval, over 350 cases were corrected by the Lillehei and Varco teams, including Dr. Aldo Castaneda and Dr. Demetre Nicoloff.

60

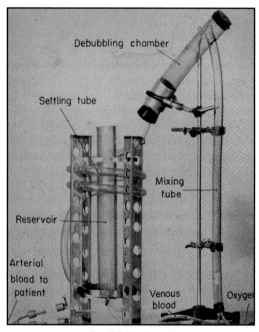

Debubbling chamber

Settling tube

Mixing tube

Reservoir

Arterial blood to patient

Venous blood

Oxyge

Dewall Bubble Oxygenator

Complications of a different nature occurred in a number of patients with ventricular septal defects (septum between the ventricles). Correction required sutures to close these defects, or be repaired with artificial plastic. The pacing mechanism of the heart was interfered with by the tight suturing of the defect and heart block ensued (rhythm abnormality). At the time of suturing the defect, unfortunately the nerves were included in the suture line and thus arrhythmias occurred and the heart stopped (heart block) and then heart failure and death followed.

At the time, an electrical engineer named Earl Bakken was repairing pressure gauges in the lab. Dr. Lillehei had already used electrodes that were sutured to the heart and an AC power source was used as the electrical system to stimulate heart activity. Dr. Lillehei and Varco used this method temporarily. Unfortunately, this source burned the heart and was poorly controlled. Eventually, the system required a 12 volt battery which was awkward and prevented patient mobility. Wires were strung across floors everywhere. It was obvious a different technique was necessary. This was emphasized when a power failure occurred during a storm and the patient's heart stopped. This was disastrous. At this point in 1958, Dr. Lillehei contacted Earl Bakken to come up with a different system. Dr. Bakken was reading a popular engineering magazine article about the electrical guts of a metronome (a music device to keep time). He studied the metronome and used basic circuitry to produce the first pacemaker (rhythm controller) to be worn on the outside of the chest.

He brought the device to the lab to test on dogs and it demonstrated to be successful. A few days later as he was walking on the cardiac surgery wards to check other monitoring systems, to his surprise he saw the same device he used on dogs the day before, being used on a human child. He questioned Dr. Lillehei who explained the patient was dying so he decided to use Dr. Bakken's experimental device. This stimulated the beginning of further development of the pacemaker. Dr. Lillehei, in his brash but genial manner followed the Wangensteen diction of lab to humans with no fuss, no committees, and an aggressive approach. Today that would be impossible.

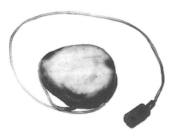

One of the first implantable pacemakers manufactured by Medtronic in 1960, with the Hunter-Roth electrode.

First Pacemaker

Meanwhile at St. Joseph Hospital in St. Paul, Minnesota Dr. Sam Hunter and Norman Roth, an engineer from Medtronic, developed a bipolar electrode which allowed the unit to be worn internally and eventually be transistorized (motorized). An electrical engineer by the name of Wilson Greatbatch (from Buffalo, NY) worked with this innovative system and collaborated with Bakken to eventually manufacture the units by the young corporation, Medtronic, Inc. These events led to the Minnesota success of the open-heart story solving the heart block problem.

Another influence on the cardiac surgery program progression was the great cardiac pathologist, Dr. Jesse Edwards, from the Mayo Clinic and later Miller Hospital in St. Paul, Minnesota where he started a heart bank. He met weekly with the cardiac teams and helped to evaluate mistakes and then correct the problems surgically. He evaluated complex anomalies and determined what it took for surgical correction, eventually started a heart bank, and taught many students in the heart program. It is obvious that many hundreds of lives have been saved, due to original experimentation by Dr. Wangensteen's students and colleagues with Wangensteen's professional influence and basic principles. Persistence in laboratory experimentation learning basic procedures with his encouragement and support, and making goals with the basic cardiac knowledge applied from the teaching of Dr. Maurice Visscher, were responsible for many incredible firsts in the heart areas. This is the Minnesota influence in the field of open-heart surgery.

Another caveat to mention was Dr. Wangensteen's keen observation. While making rounds with Dr. Walton Lillehei, then a resident in the 1940's, Dr. Wangensteen noticed a lump in front of Dr. Lillehei's right ear. He told Walt he must have this lesion biopsied. This sampling led to a diagnosis of lymphoma (lymph cancer). No adequate chemotherapy was available in those days. Dr. Wangensteen assembled a team of his trained staff to operate in a very radical fashion, knowing this tumor spreads to the head, neck and mediastinum (mid chest) as well as a local spread to the parotid gland (in front of the ear). Subsequently, Dr. Lillehei agreed to a very radical approach outlined by Dr. Wangensteen. Dr. David State carried out the parotid resection, Dr. Arnold Kremen did the radical neck dissection, and Dr. Richard Varco split the sternum and did a radical mediastinal lymph node dissection (clean out). This Wangensteen radical approach saved Dr. Walt Lillehei's life; a brilliant mind that later would become a giant in the origin of open-heart surgery.

Chapter 7
The Impact of Earl Bakken and his Associates on Cardiology and Cardiac Surgery – Coordination of Industry and Medicine

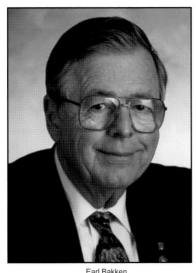

Earl Bakken

Earl Bakken was the co-founder, CEO, and Chairman Emeritus of Medtronic Inc. This is a fascinating story and having had a personal relationship with Mr. Bakken, I was intrigued with his successful progression and impact on the University of Minnesota cardiac surgery program. His leadership, perserverance, and inspiration as head of Medtronic eventually led to the company's success. Mr. Bakken was basically very interested in electronics, having been in the Armed Forces and exposed to radar in the late 1940's. Upon his return to civilian life, he was interested in electronics and enrolled in the University of Minnesota. He received a Bachelor of Science degree in electrical engineering. He started to repair malfunctioning equipment in the laboratory and, at the time, was the only individual in the area repairing the machines. He and his brother-in-law Palmer Hermundslie met in 1949 and discussed the possibility of exploring a business opportunity. Since Palmer was more of a businessman and Earl Bakken was an electronic engineer, they made a good combination. They had very few funds in the beginning, so they decided to set up an electronic medical firm.

Their first business began in a small garage owned by Palmer and his family; essentially in a used railroad car. They started out with very little capital and few jobs. Palmer handled the business and Earl handled the electronics. On April 29, 1949, they started the company called Medtronic, the combination of medicine and

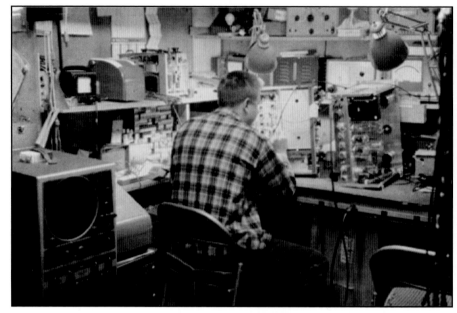

Mr. Bakken in garage office

electronics. They began stocking basic parts in Palmer's "garage" and started out by servicing electronic equipment at Abbott Hospital in Minneapolis. They also began servicing blood pressure gauges and other electronic systems at the University of Minnesota. At the startup of this company they had no sense at what it was to eventually become. They struggled for funds, but fortunately there was no rent. At first, the business progressed strictly through local hospitals and doctor's offices repairing electronic systems. Thus, they were highly specialized. In the first year, business progressed to the point where they hired one electronic technician.

In 1950, Earl Bakken visited the Sanborn Company in Boston. They manufactured electro-cardio graphic machines, pressure recorders, and other diagnostic equipment. Mr. Bakken established both selling and repairing relationships with Sanborn and later developed business with different instrument companies, such as Advanced Instruments Incorporated. Personal relationships were extremely important in the development of this area. He also began calling on hospitals and clinics in the five state area. Most important was the establishment of relationships with individuals at the University of Minnesota Hospital. Mr. Bakken's reliability paid off. Most of the electronic equipment created in the late 1950's were monitoring devices and other diagnostic, EKG, and blood flow machines. I had Earl make me an electronic flow meter I later used to measure gastric blood flow in my laboratory. This was for original work describing stress ulcer during central nervous system stimulation and required a special device. There were very few electronic therapeutic devices at the time.

During that period, cardiologists at the University Hospital and other clinics, such as the Mayo Clinic, were beginning to do some cardiac (heart) catheterizations, which were important in the diagnosis for open-heart surgery. Medtronic, under Earl's aeges, would sell them specific recorders, set up the equipment and developed close relationships with University and Mayo physicians and personnel. He was moreover, brought into the operating room and became friendly with the anesthesiologists who used a number of these instruments for monitoring anesthesia. Most of the equipment was developed and sold for the Sanborn Company. These relationships were important because in the 1950's, this led to the acquaintance with Dr. C. Walton Lillehei's group working in the laboratory and in the promising new area of open-heart surgery. He would provide them with customized recording devices used during their experimental operations. He would also troubleshoot machines and repair them.

During the mid 1950's, Dr. C. Walton Lillehei was operating on blue babies whose congenital defect produced poorly oxygenated blood. Unfortunately, during some of the operative procedures, the babies' heart conduction system, which produced electrical impulses, were surgically impaired. A defect called heart block was present. In other words, if electronic impulses stopped, the heart was not stimulated and would stop (arrest). Dr. Lillehei had used a big alternating current powered pacemaking apparatus that had come into use at the time. But it was bulky and had vacuum tubes and had to be wheeled around in a cart and plugged into the wall. I can remember as a resident, electric cords running all over the floor area which were hooked onto these AC electrical pacemaking units. These were considered state-of-the-art equipment. These units needed to be hooked up into the wall or into a twelve-volt battery. One time, during a storm, the electricity went out and the individual who was hooked up to one of these machines died. One of the original machines was developed by the group of John Callaghan, Milfred Bigelow and J.S. Hopps, who also developed a primitive pacemaker. Because of open-heart work, there was a need to develop a much more sophisticated device. At the University of Minnesota Hospitals, because the bulk of the machines and the electronic limitations of current, the effectiveness of theses devices was not the best. In fact, when the power failed they were worthless.

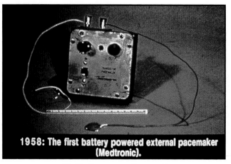

1958: The first battery powered external pacemaker (Medtronic).

First battery powered pacemaker

So, in October of 1957 after a sudden power blackout which resulted in a blue baby's loss of life, Dr. C. Walton Lillehei called Earl Bakken to see if he could come up with something more efficient for the patients. Bakken's first attempt was to have a six-volt battery converted to 115 volts of current to run the crude pacemaker. The stand was still too bulky and inefficient. In the meantime, Earl Bakken was reading an issue of Popular Electronics Magazine in which he saw the circuitry of a transistorized metronome, a device used for music rhythm monitoring, with intermittent clicks and a loudspeaker powered by a small battery. He modified the circuits and enclosed the device in a small 4 inch by 8 inch box. He had placed the battery and switches on the outside, which became the first small self-contained transistorized battery pack pacemaker. This pacemaker was then taped to the patient's chest so it freed the individual of all the cords running across the floor and the AC wall connections. The wires were to pass through the patient's chest wall, and when the pacemaker was no longer necessary, it would be removed.

The next step was more intriguing, because Dr. Bakken took the box over to the University's animal laboratory to test it out and he found out it worked quite well in animals. What was really fascinating was that the next day Earl Bakken returned to the hospital for another project. He walked past the recovery room and lo and behold he saw his experimental pacemaker used the day before on an animal, attached to one of Dr. Lillehei's patients. Earl Bakken was quite stunned and upset so he tracked down Dr. Lillehei and asked him what was going on. In Dr. Lillehei's typical no-nonsense fashion, he explained the lab personnel had told him the pacemaker worked well. He told Bakken he did not want to lose the patient so he used the pacemaker as such.

After about one month of experimentation, the world's first ever

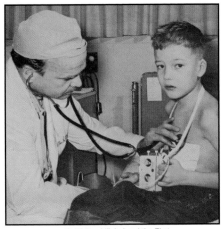

C. Walton Lillehei and the First
battery pack transistorized pacemaker

battery pack transistorized cardiac pacemaker was created, began saving lives, and started being used throughout the community. Today, a device such as this would need to go through a number of randomized prospective studies before the government and the community would accept it. As in the Wangensteen era, these individuals had foresight and experimental backup so when something worked, they used it. Bakken thus began manufacturing the device. The papers and medical community were calling it the miracle of the time. By 1958, Mr. Bakken sold about sixty of these pacemakers.

As with any other device, it became apparent innovations of the apparatus would surface. One of the most important improvements was developed by Dr. Sam Hunter of St. Joseph's Hospital in St. Paul, Minnesota and was demonstrated to Dr. Lillehei. The battery pack unit worked effectively on blue baby patients or those with injured cardiac pacing problems in the acute stage. However some adult patients had chronic progressive pacing conditions which resulted in long-term type heart block. Dr. Hunter worked with engineer Norman Roth, from Medtronic, and developed a bi-polar wiring system to the heart. This system required about three fourths less current than the original technology. The first one was implanted in 1959 in a patient who lived approximately seven years with the device.

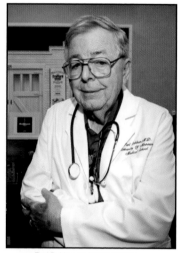

Earl Bakken as honorary M.D.

At the same time, new prototypes were being produced. In late 1958, a Swedish surgeon Dr. Ake Senning worked with an electronic engineer, Rune Elmqvist, and implanted the first internal pacemaker. The device was powered by a nickel cadmium rechargeable battery but did not last more than a few hours. Interestingly enough, a second device was designed which was considerably improved in a different way. In Buffalo, New York, Dr. William Chardack and Wilson Greatbatch, an engineer, performed animal studies to develop an implantable powered pacemaker using a battery developed in the United States. Dr. Chardack implanted them and these pioneers became friends with Earl Bakken who introduced them to the Hunter-Roth electrode. These individuals signed a significant license agreement with Bakken, and the new implantable pacemaker became the basis of manufacturing for the company of Medtronic. These pioneers, with electronic knowledge and their foresight in combination with Dr. Walt Lillehei's medical needs and encouragement were responsible for saving thousands of lives throughout the years. This is one of the great successes in cardiology and cardiac surgery. Dr. Wangensteen was very intrigued and was very encouraging to Dr. Lillehei and Mr. Bakken for this whole system. The Surgery Department at the University of Minnesota became most influential in the progress of open-heart surgery and the treatment of cardiac rhythm abnormalities. Mr. Earl Bakken received an honorary M.D. degree from the University of Minnesota for his efforts.

Chapter 8
Major Influences on the Origin of Open Heart Surgery
The Story of Dr. Jesse Edwards

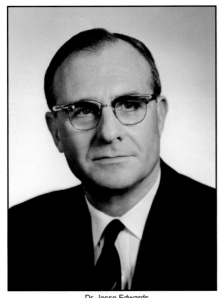
Dr. Jesse Edwards

Dr. Jesse Edwards had a major influence on open-heart surgery. He was one of the world's expert heart pathologists. He had incredible experience in reviewing cardiac pathology subsequent to death in pre and post surgery of congenital and acquired defects. He published over seven hundred twenty-five papers, interviews and articles, eleven books, and seventy chapters (the majority of which depicted pathology of heart disease).

How does this relate to cardiovascular surgery and its progressive success at the University of Minnesota hospitals? Jesse graduated from medical school in 1935 from Tufts University. He took his residency in pathology at the Mallory Institute of Pathology in Boston, Massachussetts. He was then a research fellow in 1940 at the National Cancer Institute in Bethesda, Maryland where he graduated with a crucial interest in cardiac pathology. In the 1940s, he began studying and writing about the cardiac system, its relationship to congenital anomalies and acquired heart disease, and assessing heart attack pathology. He became a Professor of Pathology in the graduate school at the University of Minnesota in 1960. This is where he generated an interest in the original heart surgery carried out by Dr. C. Walt Lillehei, Dr. Richard Varco, Dr. Aldo Castaneda and Dr. Demetre Nicoloff.

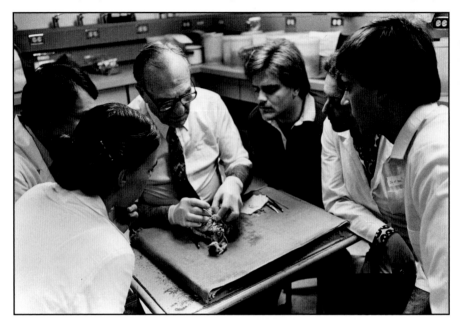

Dr. Edwards teaching residents

He had been a consultant in the section of pathology and cardiology at the Mayo Clinic in Rochester, Minnesota from 1946-1960 and Dr. John Kirklin was the cardiac surgeon. Dr. Edwards worked both at Mayo and the University of Minnesota using his vast cardiac knowledge in these blossoming programs. It was in that area in the late 1950's that he felt he could help cardiac surgeons especially at the University of Minnesota to understand the basic pathology of the heart and why some of the failures occurred following open-heart attempts in very sick pediatric cardiac patients.

It was because of his basic knowledge and understanding of the severe congenital defects that Dr. Lillehei and Dr. Varco led the way to giving a full professorship to Dr. Edwards. Dr. Edwards also started a heart bank at Miller Hospital in St. Paul, Minnesota which led to his becoming a teaching giant in cardiovascular pathology. Thus, the Dr. Jesse E. Edwards legacy in cardiovascular disease was established. He became a senior consultant of cardiovascular disease from 1960-1987 at both the University of Minnesota and Mayo Clinic. This was an important move for Dr. Edwards. He passed on his knowledge of pathology of open-hearts, by participating in open-heart surgery rounds at the University, as well as special conferences on Saturdays, in the presence of Dr. Varco, Dr. Lillehei, Dr. Demetre Nicoloff and Dr. Aldo Castaneda, as well as adult and pediatric cardiologists and residents on the cardiovascular service. It was a fascinating experience to listen to Dr. Edwards' comments and suggestions to improve techniques. It was interesting to hear the description of the complex cardiac defects that were being corrected by Dr. Varco and Dr. Lillehei, and those individuals who had followed such as Dr.

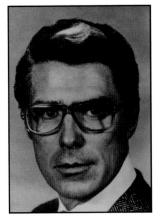

Dr. Aldo Castaneda

Demetre Nicoloff and Dr. Aldo Castaneda. He simply described the defects to the operator, what mistakes were made and how he thought these defects could be corrected. In most instances, he was absolutely right. These critiques became a mainstay in the basic understanding of early open-heart cardiac surgery on infants and individuals with severe acquired or congenital heart disease. Without the astute analysis by Dr. Edwards, many of the complex defects would not have been correctly fixed. Incidentally, his Registry of Cardiac Pathology remains as a training program for fledgling and senior cardiac surgeons even to this day and individuals come from all over the United States and all over the world to learn basic cardiac pathology to help them in surgical decision-making. Here is where "learning from mistakes" was important in improving cardiac technique.

Dr. Owen Wangensteen was intrigued by Dr. Edwards' vast knowledge. He and Dr. Edwards had a very interesting relationship. Dr. Wangensteen was very appreciative of Jesse's ability and of his help in suggesting innovations for the complex defects in infants, children, and acquired heart disease. Dr. Edwards also carried out his interests in pathology at Mayo Clinic starting in 1946. At that time period, only closed heart procedures were being carried out.

The Story of the Minnesota Influence on American Surgery

Dr. Edwards had a very perceptive mind and at Mayo he helped to understand the basic pathophysiology which occurred with these acquired defects. He understood the interior of the heart and suggested atrial and ventricular "holes in the heart" produced high blood pressure in the lungs. He predicted some sort of open-heart closure would be needed to correct and prevent the pressure defect.

The correction at the University of Minnesota as the first open-heart procedure in the world was an atrial septal defect (hole in the atrial system) in 1952 by Dr. F. John Lewis and Dr. Richard Varco under hypothermia or cooling the body. Only five minutes was available to correct the defect by this method. Following this event with the advent of the cross circulation and the pump oxygenator several of the septal defects in the atrium and the ventricle as predicted by Dr. Edwards, caused problems in pulmonary flow that could not be dealt with unless open-heart surgery correction was carried out. Also, complex defects involving the valves and transposition (reversing) of the great vessels and single ventricles, as examples, required longer times at surgery, which was provided by the pump oxygenator to correct these defects. Once the pump oxygenator was developed, Dr. Edwards' work became both important and necessary in understanding the basic pathology of the heart. This is where Dr. Edwards' heart book and his pathology bank helped advance the surgery of these complex defects. Thus, open-heart surgery was advanced at the University of Minnesota and the Mayo Clinic as the surgeons learned the pathophysiology from Dr. Edwards. Dr. Brooks Edwards (son of Dr. Jesse Edwards) and Dr. James Moller, both cardiologists at Mayo Clinic and the University of Minnesota respectively, recently published an excellent summary of Dr. Edwards' accomplishments.

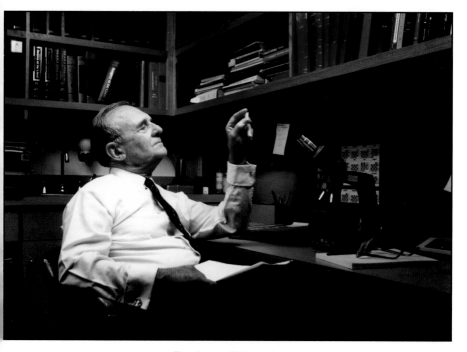

Dr. Jesse Edwards

Chapter 9
Colo-Rectal Surgery Division

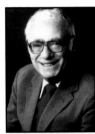

Dr. William Bernstein

The colorectal division at the University of Minnesota is, at present, one of the leading training centers of its kind in the United States. Its origin had a rather auspicious and fascinating beginning with credit given to Dr. Wangensteen and Dr. William Bernstein.

In an interview with Dr. Bernstein, it became apparent a typical approach of encouragement was exhibited by Dr. Wangensteen in what was then a primitive field (1930's). This relationship became the basis for one of the first large diagnostic, therapeutic and training proctology divisions of surgery.

Dr. Bernstein interned in 1927 at Anker Hospital (now Regions Hospital). He entered private practice in New Richmond, Wisconsin with encouragement from Dr. William Peyton, then a neurosurgeon at the University of Minnesota. In 1936, he was bored with practice and decided to go into the surgical specialty of proctology. Dr. Fansler, who was practicing proctology in Minneapolis at that time, informed Dr. Bernstein there was no residency in this specialty at the University but if one was started, Dr. Bernstein would be the first resident. By 1939, there was no residency forthcoming, since there was no specialty board in that discipline as of yet. Dr. Bernstein enrolled in the graduate school as a voluntary resident and proceeded to take basic courses in anatomy, pathology, and physiology. His surgical experiences in proctology were with Dr. Fansler, who was the "director" of the yet to be specialty. In 1939 he asked Dr. Fansler to notify Dr. Wangensteen of his plans and Dr. Bernstein started working at the University hospital on January 2, 1940. One day, he went to the outpatient clinic and found a note from Dr. Wangensteen asking to see him. Dr. Wangensteen told Dr. Bernstein he had heard he was enrolled as a graduate student in the Department of Surgery. He told Dr. Bernstein he, Dr. Wangensteen, was the Chairman of the department and not Dr. Fansler. Any arrangements he made in the

Through The Portals of Pigs and Manure

Department of Surgery would be made with Dr. Wangensteen, not Dr. Fansler. Dr. Wangensteen did, however, manifest an interest in Dr. Bernstein's program and asked to see him in a few months when he was more confident in diagnostics and techniques in that time specialty. Dr. Bernstein returned in September of 1940.

In June 1940, an incident occurred and brought things to a head. Dr. Wangensteen's resident on purple surgery (Dr. Wangensteen's surgery service) placed a rectal tube in a patient and fastened it in place with a suture. The patient had a partial obstruction and was supposed to have soapsuds enemas twice a day as a treatment regimen. After this solution was administered, the fluid did not return. The tube had eroded the rectum and perforated the bowel. The patient was emergently operated on, the perforation closed and he survived. Dr. Bernstein saw Dr. Wangensteen to report the problem and thought his fate was sealed. However, Dr. Wangensteen was most considerate and generous. He did not think Dr. Bernstein was to fault. Instead, he blamed his chief resident, suggesting the tube should have been moved every twenty four hours to prevent such an occurrence. He then inquired of Dr. Bernstein's progress and suggested he start rectal surgery in the operating room at the University Hospital. In 1942, he called Dr. Bernstein and said he knew very little about common rectal operations and suggested Dr. Bernstein be his alter ego and take care of patients with these conditions in the future.

Dr. Bernstein practiced rectal surgery in St. Paul, Minnesota and ran the outpatient rectal program at the University Hospital instructing the interns and residents. Unfortunately, he was called into the Army in 1943, returning in 1946. Upon his return, Dr. Wangensteen asked Dr. Bernstein to start his own clinic at the University on Thursdays. This was occasioned by the fact that when Dr. Bernstein was away, one of his private patients was proctoscoped by another physician and was told he had a negative exam up to the twenty five cm level. The patient died several days later. At post mortem, the patient had perforated a cancer at the fifteen cm level. From that moment on, Dr. Wangensteen was emphatic only Dr. Bernstein would proctoscope his patients. Dr. Bernstein's relationship with Dr. Wangensteen was cordial for a long time. However, he received a critical letter asking why he was not available on a Tuesday to scope one of his patients. Dr. Bernstein reminded Dr. Wangensteen he had made the arrangement for a Thursday scope day. Dr. Wangensteen apologized in a letter, a rare gesture by the "Chief."

By 1948, Dr. Bernstein had developed a large rectal surgery service at the US Veterans Hospital and Anker Hospital (now Regions Hospital) as well as the University Hospital. Dr. Bernstein asked for Dr. Wangensteen's permission to start a residency program combining those three facilities and his downtown practice. Dr. Wangensteen was agreeable to the suggestion. He called a meeting at the Campus Club, which included Dr. Varco, who at that time was the executive of the University surgery training program, Dean Diehl, Dr. Clarence Dennis, Dr. Fansler and Dr. Bernstein. The Dean asked if there was a certified board for the trainees. He was told a board was being organized but was not yet achieved. The meeting was adjourned to be reconvened when board status was available.

In 1949, the Board of Proctology was established and another meeting was held and permission for a program was granted. One hour after the meeting, Dr. Bernstein received a call from Dr. Wangensteen's secretary, Miss Jacobsen, stating there were no funds to support the residency program and before Dr. Bernstein started the program, funds were necessary. Within a few months, a friend of Dr. Bernstein, David Paper, agreed to support the residency.

Moreover, an incident occurred a few months later which was typical of Dr. Wangensteen. Mr. Paper needed a nephrectomy (removal of a kidney). He was at Miller Hospital in St. Paul, Minnesota. The family was alarmed after finding out the patient's BUN was 105 (nitrogen products excreted by the kidney - normal values are ten to fifteen). Dr. Bernstein called Dr. Wangensteen to ask if he would look at Mr. Paper. He did. He asked to see Mr. Paper's tongue and suggested he was very dry. Dr. Wangensteen said he relied on exam more than the laboratory tests. After treatment with several liters of fluid, the patient recovered, his kidney function returned and Dr. Wangensteen was given full credit. Mr. Paper told Dr. Bernstein he never received a bill from Dr. Wangensteen. Dr. Wangensteen told Mr. Paper he was grateful for what he had done for the University, however, he would appreciate more contributions for research. Mr. Paper sent Dr. Wangensteen a $10,000 check for research. Over time that figure reached $100,000 This was typical of Dr. Wangensteen's approach.

On another occasion, Dr. Wangensteen needed $5,000 for a specific project. He called Dave Paper who said he could easily raise the amount. Dr. Wangensteen said if that was the case, he would like $50,000, which was successfully raised.

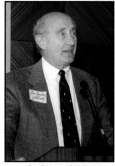

Dr. Stanley Goldberg

In any event, Dr. Bernstein was the instigator of the colo-rectal program at the University of Minnesota with encouragement from Dr. Wangensteen. This program later came under the able direction of Dr. Stanley Goldberg after Dr. Bernstein retired. Dr. Goldberg was responsible for growing his program into one of the most prolific and successful residencies in the United States. It is now a full-time division at the University. Upon Dr. Goldberg's retirement, the division came under the direction of Dr. David Rothenberger. Several division heads throughout the country have been trained in this discipline through this very successful residency program. Thus, this specialty was born at the University with Dr. Wangensteen's support and moreover, is responsible for eventual development of services throughout the country.

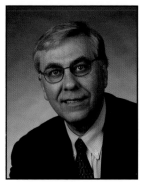

Dr. David Rothenberger

Chapter 10
Morbid Obesity Problem

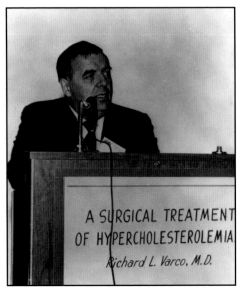
Dr. Richard Varco

The childhood obesity problem has grown to an intolerable rate. This problem has been fueled by stress, the economy, fast food company advertising, psychological, and possibly gene-based conditions. It is obvious that what is taken in as food is the common denominator. Fat contains nine calories per gram; carbohydrate and protein contain four calories per gram. The type of fat consumed and the resulting obesity also promotes several conditions including hypertension, heart problems, diabetes, pulmonary sleep apnea, and asthma.

Dr. Richard Varco and Dr. Henry Buchwald recognized these problems early in the 1960's and were pioneers in the field. With the encouragement of Dr. Wangensteen, experiments were carried out to bypass three quarters of the intestine, the jejuno ileal bypass. This experimental operation eventually led to a large series on morbid obese patients. Although good weight loss was observed, over time the procedure was abandoned due to several complications. These included liver failure, bacteriode infection in the bypassed loop, loss

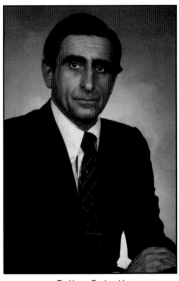
Dr. Henry Buchwald

79

of minerals from diarrhea, impaired nutrients from malabsorption, and anemia. Thus, the early weight loss resulting from the bypass, gradually was replaced with a number of problems. Over the years Dr. Buchwald then switched to gastric (stomach) bypass where a large portion of the stomach (75-80%) is bypassed by excluding it with a stapling procedure. Patients are thus forced to eat less. In experienced hands this operation has held up in morbid obese individuals. Careful preoperative evaluation and dietary trials are carried out before surgery is instituted. Effects of surgery include the lowering of blood pressure, a decrease in cholesterol, a decrease in insulin requirements in diabetes, and improvement in sleep apnea. Dr. Buchwald has continuously improved the lives of many of these individuals who are morbidly obese. His clinics and procedures and basic understanding of these morbidly obese patients were passed on to many fledgling house officers.

Obviously, exercise and diet discretion remain the basis for prevention of obesity, starting in schools. This is another Wangensteen experimental based problem brought to clinical trials with eventual improvement of quality of life and longevity.

Chapter 11
Najarian and Transplantation

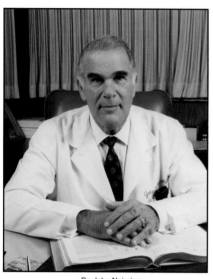

Dr. John Najarian

Dr. John Najarian from the University of California Berkley was recruited for the department head position at the University of Minnesota upon Dr. Wangensteen's retirement in 1967. This was because of his basic work in transplantation and his ability to organize. By the late 1960's, Dr. Robert Good and Dr. Richard Varco were eager to start a transplant program at the University of Minnesota. Dr. Good was a brilliant immunologist and pediatrician at the University. He understood the immune system and helped study basic immunology and designed the first bone marrow transplant at the University of Minnesota. The University also had an excellent group of pediatric nephrologists (experts in kidney disease) headed by Dr. Al Michael and Dr. Robert Vernier. Kidney transplantation had already been carried out by Dr. Joe Murray at the Peter Brent Brigham Hospital (Harvard based) in 1954, on identical twins. The transplant operation on identical twins was performed at the University of Minnesota by Dr. Richard Varco, Dr. William Kelly, Dr. Joseph Aust, and myself in 1963. Identical twins have the same gene complex and therefore accept the organ without rejection. The problem is the use of non-related donors where organs are rejected unless the immune system of the recipient is treated.

Therefore, the big problem which needed to be solved in transplantation was the rejection phenomena – where the non-related individual's organ would be rejected due to the recipient's immune response to that donor organ. The original work by Dr. Joseph Murray using radiation and an immune blocking drug called Imuran opened

81

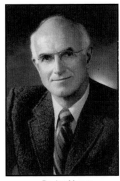

Dr. Joe Murray

the field for transplantation. Dr. Murray received the Nobel Prize in medicine for his original experimentation and implementation by the means of altering the immune response so the recipients would accept the organs even though they were not related. In 1962, Dr. Tom Starzl, from Denver, used Prednisone and Imuran to reduce the rejection phenomenon and was also a pioneer in adult liver and kidney transplantation.

Dr. Goodman at UC Berkley had already added Prednisone to Imuran to set the stage for reducing rejection. Also, Dr. Roy Calne in Cambridge, England was working on a new drug called Cyclosporine for anti-rejection as early as 1978. This drug later would replace the Imuran Prednisone combination because of less complications and better anti-rejection response.

Dr. Najarian had also carried out basic experiments in transplantation at UC San Diego, and applied them clinically when he moved to University of California Berkley from 1963-1967. He at the time successfully performed several kidney transplants. He organized a team of nephrologists who improved renal dialysis (a method to remove back-up impurities from the blood in failed kidneys). He employed a brilliant nephrologist, Dr. Carl Schelstrand from Sweden, and a young, bright and aggressive surgical staff member, Dr. Richard Simmons, as part of his team. Dr. Good, who was head of the selection committee for the appointment of a

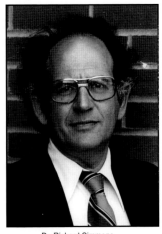

Dr. Richard Simmons

Surgery Department head upon Dr. Wangensteen's retirement, was very impressed with Dr. Najarian's progress in transplantation. He not only had a basic understanding of the rejection problem, he was an excellent organizer and surgeon. Dr. Najarian, also during his visit to Minnesota, was impressed with Dr. Wangensteen's unique training system for producing academic surgeons. He was moreover

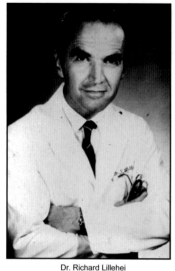
Dr. Richard Lillehei

stimulated by the presence of pediatric nephrologists Dr. Al Michael, Dr. Robert Vernier, and Dr. Robert Good's basic work in immunology.

The foundation was set for implantation of a basic transplantation program. Before Dr. Najarian's appointment, Dr. William Kelly and Dr. Richard Lillehei had already begun kidney and pancreas transplantation in adults with non-related donors. Dr. William Kelly did the first pancreas transplant at the University on December 16, 1966. Dr. Richard Lillehei did the second pancreas transplant December 31, 1966. He did twelve more pancreas transplants up to 1973.

In 1967, Dr. Najarian foresaw the progress which could ensue with a program already started with Dr. Wangensteen's approval and support and accepted the position as head of surgery. He had big shoes to fill, but "Big John" had the ingredients and the shoe size (he had been an excellent athlete, playing football at the University of California San Francisco, under the direction of Pappy Waldorf). Upon his arrival, Najarian evaluated not only the transplant program, but also the basic surgery system created by Dr. Wangensteen.

The next big step by Dr. Najarian was to improve the fight against the rejection phenomenon. Although Imuran and Prednisone were a great advance, enough rejection was present to suggest new studies be indicated. The drug Cyclosporine was not yet FDA approved.

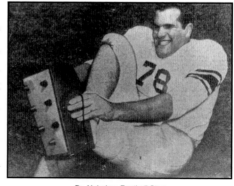
Dr. Najarian, Football Star

Through The Portals of Pigs and Manure

By 1968, Dr. Alan Moberg, in Najarian's laboratory, was already working on a new concept using a system to create anti-lymphocyte globulin to stem the rejection phenomenon. Human blood from recipient was injected into horses and a product called ALG (anti-lymphocyte globulin) was extracted. By 1969, these experiments were quite impressive. Dr. Richard Condie came in Dr. Najarian's lab, refined the technique and purified the substance so it could be given intravenously. The FDA approved the system and trials were successful without the complications of the Imuran Prednisone usage. This was a great contribution to the transplant field by Dr. Najarian and his colleagues and was used for twenty two years (see ALG problem).

The next step by Dr. Najarian that was implemented in the late 1960's and early 1970's was to start the first kidney transplant program in children with diabetes or other severe kidney problems. A group of children who had juvenile onset diabetes with resulting kidney failure were transplanted. With the team of Dr. Al Michael and Dr. Robert Vernier, pediatric nephrologists, renal transplantation flourished. Several hundred renal transplants in children were performed. Under the direction of Dr. Richard Simmons, a transplant training program, which included these children as patients was started. A postgraduate program resulted in the training of several hundred surgeons in the field from around the United States, and the world. This program became the premiere transplant training system in the United States. Now that renal transplantation flourished, attention was directed to pancreas and liver transplantation and eventually the heart. By 1980 to 1984, Cyclosporine was eventually approved and was a great improvement to stemming major rejection problems and added to the success of Dr. Najarian's approach.

Pancreas transplantation was still a problem in the late 1960's and early 1970's. Although Dr. Richard Lillehei had performed twelve pancreas transplants by 1973, the complication rate was still high even with the use of ALG (anti-lymphocyte globulin). Patients did get partial insulin relief but the surgery was quite morbid. Dr. Najarian ordered Dr. Lillehei to stop complete pancreas transplants.

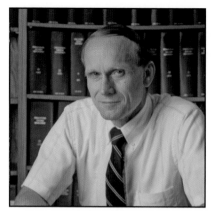

Dr. David Sutherland

Meanwhile, Dr. David Sutherland who worked in Dr. Richard Lillehei's laboratory, progressed rapidly in the University system and entered Dr. Najarian's program. In the laboratory he worked out a novel system of islet transplantation. The islets of the pancreas are cells that produce insulin. His basic laboratory work led to being hired by Dr. Najarian to head the pancreas program. By his brilliant laboratory work where he performed partial pancreas resections in animals, he developed a technique by which the islet cells were procured and injected into the portal vein (the vein leading to the liver) in animals. The transplanted islets attached to the liver cells, then to the liver tissue and lived on the blood supply to the liver and secreted insulin. The loss of insulin producing cells is the basis for the disease of diabetes. This was a way to produce insulin with a partial resection of the pancreas, using islet cells for diabetic response, not the more complicated complete pancreas resection and whole organ transplantation. This pancreas could be procured from donors or, in some instances, from the patient's own organ by partial resection and the cells then procured by the Sutherland method and subsequently given to the diabetic patient.

Dr. Sutherland carried out the first islet transplant in 1974. ALG was used to suppress rejection. After several transplants, it was apparent complete insulin independence was not gained, yet the amount of insulin necessary for these diabetic patients had significantly improved. All of these patients already had kidney transplants, thus were on immunosuppression therapy.

The next step by Dr. Najarian and Dr. Sutherland was auto transplant where instead of using donor transplanted pancreas, a partial or whole pancreas was used from the diabetic patient. Dr. Sutherland carried out the first procedure in 1977. Then, in 1978, pancreatic

Through The Portals of Pigs and Manure

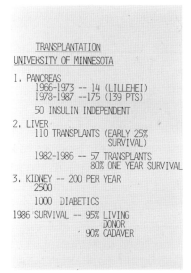

Transplantation, University of Minnesota

tissue was removed and islet cells procured and given back to the same patient (auto transplant). Therefore, rejection was averted. Also, by 1986, pancreatic transplants in diabetics were carried out in combination with kidney transplants, or alone before or after kidney transplantation. By this time, Cyclosporine, a new transplant drug, was available and used to suppress rejection. This drug made a big difference in reducing the rejection phenomenon.

In 1963 Dr. Tom Starzyl first carried out a liver transplantation on an adult. Liver failure from cirrhosis and/or hepatitis were the disease problems which were first transplanted. Later, patients with liver tumors and no apparent spread were subjected to transplantation. At first, Imuran and Prednisone were used for anti-rejection. Later, Cyclosporine was used and made a marked improvement in patient survival and quality of life. Children's liver transplants had not yet been carried out.

Najarian performed the first of several successful liver transplants at the University of Minnesota on small

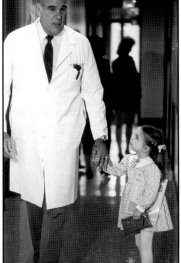

Dr. Najarian with Jamie Fiske (first liver transplant)

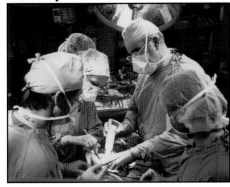

Dr. Najarian and Dr. Asher (first liver transplant in child)

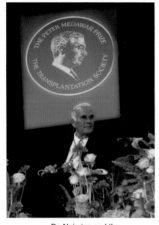

Dr. Najarian and the
Medawar Medal Ceremony

children. The first one was on Jamie Fiske. Liver transplantation then flourished at the University of Minnesota under the direction of Dr. John Najarian. Over 110 liver transplants have been performed. Patient survival improved each year. One out of every four transplants survived in 1982. After 1982 and over the next several years, fifty seven liver transplants were carried out with an 80% survival rate. The use of Cyclosporine, a new anti-rejection drug, contributed greatly to the transplant program at the University of Minnesota. Dr. Najarian trained several surgeons around the world and in the United States with his technique, using ALG for anti-rejection. He received the Medawar Prize from the Transplant Society (their highest award).

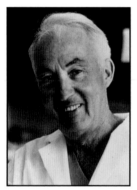

Dr. Shumway

Heart transplantation was the next bold move and began with the basic laboratory work by Dr. Norman Shumway, Dr. C. Walton Lillehei and Dr. Lawler of West Virginia University (a later colleague of Dr. Shumway). Dr. Shumway was a trainee of Dr. Wangensteen and Dr. C. Walt Lillehei. The first heart transplant was performed by Christiaan Barnard in 1967 and Dr. Shumway a few months later. Many centers tried heart transplantation, but it took teams of cardiologists and immunologists to be successful. Drs. Shumway and Lawler's original laboratory work were responsible for positive early results. Adding Cyclosporine to the transplant patients helped in the reduction of rejection (see chapter six, The Heart Story).

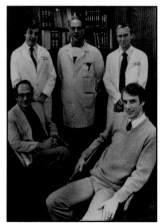

Dr. Najarian and Dr. Simmons
and the transplant group

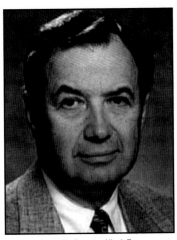
Dr. Demetre Nicoloff

In Minnesota, Dr. Demetre Nicoloff carried out the first heart transplant at the University. He continued the program at Abbott Northwestern Hospital, in Minneapolis, after he left the University. After 1980, Cyclosporine again was used in heart transplants and was responsible for repression of rejection. ALG was utilized in the early transplants as well as a combination of Imuran and Prednisone.

The centers with experienced teams had the best results, as learned and implemented by Dr. Najarian and his colleagues. These systems were all supported by basic laboratory experimentation, the hallmark of the Wangensteen and Najarian philosophy which contributed so much to the Minnesota influence on American surgery.

Chapter 12
The ALG Problem – Organ Rejection After Transplantation

One of the problems with transplantation of the kidney, pancreas, liver or any transplanted organ, is the inconsistency of the phenomena called rejection. The body's immune system ramps up when it sees a foreign organ placed in it and tries to destroy the organ. Dr. Najarian was interested in improving the ability of the body to accept transplanted organs without creating rejection, a form of inflammation that eventually dismantles the organ's ability to perform it's normal function.

A scientist, Sir Michael Woodruff from Scotland, worked with an anti-lymphocyte serum and reported increased survival in rat skin grafts. This experimental report caught Dr. Najarian's interest and kindled the beginning of research at the University of Minnesota and eventual production of what is called anti-lymphocyte globulin serum (ALG) which reduces the immune effects on the transplanted organ.

In 1964, Dr. Iwasakai of the University of Colorado began, with support of Dr. Tom Starzl, an eminent transplant surgeon, to produce ALG by injecting human cells into horses and collecting the serum to use in transplanted patients. The horses' immune systems reacted to the cells by producing ALG. The Colorado group was the first to use this early type serum in patients receiving kidney transplants. The rejection phenomenon was partially affected. Unfortunately, the pain present during muscle injection, the only way it was given, was severe plus the body eventually rejected the serum.

Dr. Najarian was inspired by the problem and began research at the University under the direction at first by Dr. Allen Moberg, one of the surgery residents in his laboratory. Instead of using inconsistent patient serum lymphocytes, a method was developed to grow human lymphocytes in culture. This led to a much more consistent production by the horses of the anti-lymphocyte globulin, the substance produced by the horse immune system to eventually ward off rejection in patients' transplanted organs. However, the process needed to be purified and Dr. Richard Condie, an immunologist who in the past had studied under the direction of Dr. Robert Good (a brilliant University of Minnesota immunologist), was lured from Roosevelt Hospital in New York to Minnesota to purify the ALG. Survival rates of experimentally transplanted organs improved by 15-20%. FDA approval was granted to manufacture, recover costs and use ALG. For twenty two years, the ALG serum was used and manufactured at the University of Minnesota. In a randomized clinical study, it was demonstrated the ALG produced by the Minnesota group was as effective as the Imuran Prednisone combination and Cyclosporine, a newer anti-rejection drug, without serious side effects. In a human study by Halloran et al. from Canada ALG was deemed the safest. As a result, the Minnesota product gained scientific popularity and was used in many transplant centers and saved many transplanted organs.

At this point, a pharmaceutical company competitively manufacturing a different type of ALG complained to the FDA about unfair competition. Also, a leaking bottle containing ALG was found in a San Diego hospital and was reported to the FDA. In addition, some deaths in these very sick patients were not reported to the FDA with the possible cause by ALG. These incidents resulted in the shut down of the Minnesota program despite the fact that over 60,000 patients were treated with the serum. The shut down in 1992 was after twenty two years of experience with great success in preventing the rejection reaction.

From that point on, a variety of investigations by the NIH, FDA, and FBI were undertaken and various charges were brought against Dr. Najarian and his manufacturing program. Despite the approval of the FDA to manufacture and recover costs, charges piled up. Over the next four years and in a trial in 1996, Dr. Najarian proved he received no personal benefit, and the nine death cases the government claimed were not reported because the deaths were not due to ALG. Dr. Najarian also proved the drug was legally being sold. Also, letters of approval by the FDA were produced to support legality of manufacturing and the recovery of costs.

The human blow to Dr. Najarian was compounded by non-support from the University, even after he had developed such a great transplant program that undoubtedly saved thousands of lives. In January of 1996 at the final ALG trial, Judge Kyle's decision was in favor of Dr. Najarian after examination of all the facts. However, Dr. Najarian had already, by order of the University, lost his departmentship head. This move by the University created furor among many academic surgeons throughout the transplant and surgery community, the fact that the University would not back its own productive person.

In a move by Peter Thompson, Dr. Najarian's attorney, letters were sent to Dr. Frank Cerra, Vice President of Medical Affairs, and Dr. Alfred Michael, Dean of the Medical School, to provide a Chair in Dr. Najarian's name in the field of transplantation as a conciliatory gesture to him. All agreed and eventually the Chair was funded by many of "Big John's" close, loyal friends in the field of transplantation. This is one of the highest honors provided by the University to its recipient. Also, a yearly endowed transplantation lectureship in John's name was awarded to him by the Department of Surgery. John certainly deserved these awards, especially after developing one of the great transplant training centers in the world. What a toll on Dr. Najarian's life, expended funds, and loss of a proven effective drug for helping to counteract the rejection of transplanted organs. Certainly Dr. Najarian is one of the great transplant surgeons of our time. He had a great influence on American surgery not only by developing a world class training transplant program, but by many firsts in transplantation including kidney transplantation in diabetic children and liver transplants in children with end stage liver disease.

Chapter 13
John Najarian and Academic Surgery

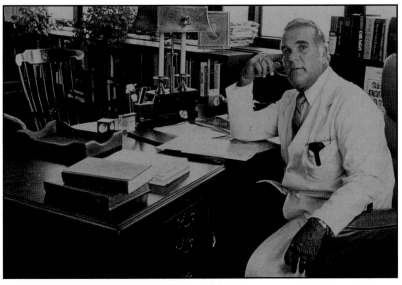

Dr. John Najarian

After entering the Surgery Department as head in 1967, Dr. Najarian looked at the overall residency program in order to improve the clinical surgery component. Under the leadership of Dr. Owen H. Wangensteen, residents were placed in a variety of different clinical schedules and laboratory time. The program was too variable. The trainee might go to the lab for one, two or even three years directly after internship. Some would have a year or two of junior clinical training before laboratory. After their laboratory training, they would emerge as senior resident on a clinical service, then became chief resident. In many instances, they were deficient in many aspects of clinical problems both diagnostic and technical. Dr. Wangensteen felt the laboratory should provide much training in the way of surgical technique. To improve the surgical clinical experience, and make a more uniform approach, Dr. Najarian made some very significant alliances with Dr. Ed Humphrey at Vets Hospital, Dr. Earl Yanehiro at Methodist Hospital, and Dr. John Perry at Ramsey General Hospital in St. Paul (now Regions Hospital). In each area, significant clinical training was added to the surgery program. Senior residents would spend quality time with advanced surgeons. The trauma program at Regions Hospital gave a well-rounded addition to the program. Over the years, attempts to provide emergency training at Minneapolis General (now Hennepin County Medical Center) failed to be added for more trauma experience. Dr. Claude Hitchcock maintained that his institution was independent from the University. I believe that because Dr. Owen H. Wangensteen did not keep him on the staff, he was disappointed and remained independent from the University program. Instead, trauma training was added to the training program at North Memorial Hospital.

Residents were delighted with these experiences. By 1969 or 1970, all of these rotations were added to the program and thus improved the clinical abilities of the academic trained surgeons. Dr. Wangensteen had also established what is known as "complication conferences." At this meeting, residents would explain mistakes made in their surgical endeavors for the week and stand on their own for explanations. Criticism would be forthcoming from staff and other residents. Technical questions were also discussed. Thus, there was a free dynamic discussion by all. Constructive remarks were mostly adopted, sometimes in heated responses. This freedom of individual response was the hallmark of sessions, far different from many discussions in the other departments in the country, with limited free response. Dr. Najarian retained this program.

Another conference which we all participated in was Saturday Grand Rounds, where a subject was presented and opinions were sometimes emotionally voiced. All levels of participants including division heads, the "Chief," residents, interns and students were equally participating in the discussions. This session was a far cry from many of the east coast departments where the head had the last word. These were great surgical learning experiences for all. Dr. Najarian kept these conferences for obvious reasons.

Another area where "Big John" contributed to the education of not only our residents and students was that of a yearly continuation course given for accreditation for surgical education to surgeons locally and around the country. Experts in several fields such as GI, breast, endocrine, vascular and trauma were invited from around the country to participate and educate about their expertise. Several hundred participants from around the country and world enjoyed these sessions. Dr. John Delaney teamed with Dr. Najarian to implement these programs.

Dr. Najarian was the second "great" to head our department. In his ensuing four decades, the academic training department was kept alive and thriving, training in his period as "Chief" over 200 academic surgeons (twenty as department chairmen, fifty as division heads in various disciplines). Also, over 100 transplant academic trainees of his are spread throughout the United States and around the world. This is quite a legacy to be proud of, with great impact on surgery in the United States and around the world. Dr. Wangensteen and Dr. Najarian were two of the most prolific educators and producers of academic surgeons in the country. By solving laboratory problems and creating well-rounded clinical services, students and residents were able to query the unknown and be better equipped to solve clinical problems.

Owen H. Wangensteen's program, with 100 residents and 100 beds has been a mystery throughout the surgical academic world. Other surgical programs have proposed several questions and the deans of many medical schools have wondered where the money for these trainees came from. From his inception as "Chief," Wangensteen in many instances did not charge his patients. Instead, he would suggest they give a contribution to his research fund. Over the years, millions of dollars have been raised to support his program. In the early years of 1930 to the late 1950's, John Hopkins' program under the aegis of Dr. William Halsted , "The Father of American Surgery", was an eight or nine year program. This system was for the most part clinically oriented in contrast to the Wangensteen program which was heavily involved in a research oriented system. This program was responsible for the many innovative advances in intestinal obstruction, cardiac surgery, transplantation, ulcer reforms, and the pacemaker, to name a few. Wangensteen's program was the main stimulus which attracted John Najarian to follow in Dr. Wangensteen's footsteps. Dr. Najarian certainly had the "big feet" to step right in to the program to add many improvements as well as begin a world-class transplant program.

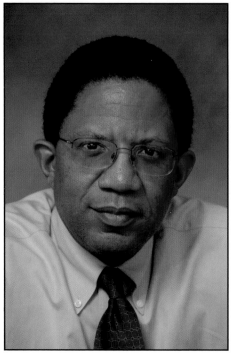

Dr. Seldon Vickers

After Najarian stepped down, Ed Humphrey, from the Veterans Hospital temporarily ran the department from 1983-1984 until Dr. David Dunn was appointed head of the department. Dr. Dunn had done a great deal of basic primary work in bacteriology and endotoxin work and had a number of residents in his lab. He left the University in 2005 and Dr. Seldon Vickers was then appointed chairman of the department. He did his basic work in pancreatic tumor work, has a very calm personality, and is well liked by residents. He is a good administrator, and gets along well with administration. He believes in parity between the divisions. He also appointed Dr. Ashok Fraluja as head of the laboratories working on new treatments for pancreatic cancer. He is very interested in continuing the academic and experimental programs established by his predecessors Dr. Wangensteen and Dr. Najarian.

Chapter 14
Whale Surgery: A First and a Challenge

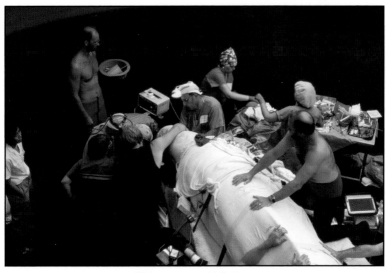

Whale on operating table for biopsy

I was called by the Minnesota Zoo staff veterinarian, Dr. Frank Wright, regarding a problem with Big Mouth, a 1700 pound beluga whale. Big Mouth had a painful ulcerating lesion on the lower jaw expanding and interfering with his ability to maintain nutrition. For two years the lesion progressed despite antibiotic treatment. The first question was what was the pathology of the lesion? Was it infection or a tumor? A biopsy was necessary. I was called because of my experience with reconstruction. No one had ever operated on a whale, so a task force was assembled to assess risks and indications. I was asked to head a seventeen member team including anesthesiologists, nurses, veterinarian support, ENT and maxillary specialist surgeons to biopsy the area. An advisory panel of ocean/marine

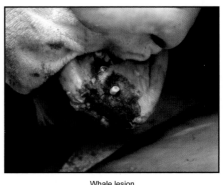

Whale lesion

The Story of the Minnesota Influence on American Surgery

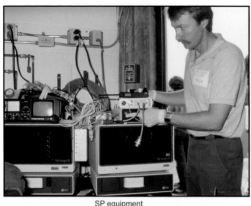
SP equipment

specialists from zoos around the country, an EKG whale specialist from Sweden, pathologists, and University Veterinarian School experts all met on May 28, 1986. Risks were discussed. Many members voiced opposition to surgery. Ron Tilson, Division Director of Biologic Programs, stated that without surgery, Big Mouth would not live in his present, deteriorating status. I felt we had three alternatives. If Big Mouth, who had been hand-fed for years, was placed at sea, he would not live. If nothing was done, the mammal would starve from pain and inability to orally take nutrition, and die from infection. The only real alternative was surgical correction of the deformity on the lower jaw, once a diagnosis was obtained. Finally, the panel agreed. A biopsy was set for June 19, 1986. Dr. Frank Wright from the zoo veterinarian team was responsible for assembling the zoo personnel and operating facility. Veterinary anesthesiologists and pathologists were informed of the procedure. We adopted a Mayon tubing to a bird respirator to place in the blowhole for oxygen administration, and respiration. Just as a human, the mammal was monitored by EKG, oxygen, CO2, and chemistries at short intervals during surgery by previously placed arterial and venous catheters. Intravenous fluids were calculated by weight. The animal was lowered by crane onto an operating table constructed of wood and polystyrene. Oxygen was administered through the whale's blowhole to maintain oxygen saturation and carbon dioxide stability. Anesthesia was administered locally. The sedation drugs Marcaine, Demerol, and Valium (a tranquilizer) were given intravenously. Blood pressure was monitored. Dr. Norman Berlinger, Associate Professor of ENT, and Dr. Lawrence Marenette, Director of maxilla facial reconstruction at Hennepin County Medical Center, assisted me in the full thickness biopsy procedure.

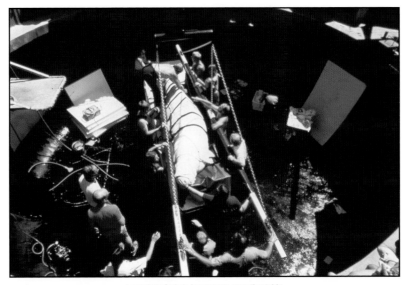

Lowering of whale by crane to operating table

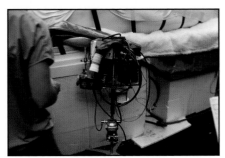

Modified bird respirator, local anethesia
prior to excision of mandible

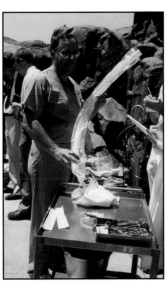

Mayon tubing for blowhole

This procedure served as a tune-up for the extensive mandible resection scheduled for July 10, 1986. Biopsy was carried out with good blood control and the area reconstructed with mouth tissue to prevent further blood loss. Results revealed an infectious process, aggressive and destroying the mandible, thus responsible for excess pain. Skeptics of any surgery were happy with this "extraordinary" initial challenge. The volunteer whale team was delighted. The duplicated monitoring as in humans worked well. I received several cards from children who were whale friends cheering us on to save the whale. The next step was the big procedure where a mandible partial resection was scheduled for July 10, 1986. We assembled our team of nurses from the University, operating room equipment, and suture material for wound closure, including heavy wire and strong teflac nylon type sutures. The above specialist physicians were summoned to assist in this groundbreaking challenge. After local and systemic drug anesthesia was administered and monitoring catheters and EKG applied, the blowhole was intubated and oxygen administered with the aid of the modified bird respirator. We had previously examined a whale mandible, sent from the Chicago Zoo, to study the anatomy, and to help us gain blood control. We used large antibiotic containing capsules to prevent excess blood loss by plugging the large openings in the jaw where vessels resided. After the whale was anesthetized locally, teeth were removed and the mandible lesion was excised with an oscillating saw.

Once the lesion was removed, reconstruction with wires, screws, and advancement of skin flaps left Big Mouth with an "Andy Gump" look (recessed lower jaw). The operation went well with good blood and pain control. The blood was replaced with large amounts of IV fluids. The complete surgical team including the veterinarian staff, performed very well. The zoo group deserves a great deal of credit for the preoperative and postoperative preparations in the whale. The jaw portion removed was seven inches wide, five inches long, and four inches deep. Wound checks were carried out weekly. The large reconstruction wire sutures were removed four weeks later and the wound healed well. The whale immediately started eating several pounds of fish daily. It was a very emotional experience when Big Mouth was placed into a large tank holding Little Girl, his female companion. He immediately penetrated her. Following recovery, I felt the whales should be sent to Sea World in San Diego, California where natural ocean water would be available and increase the chance for long-term survival. Both whales were sent in large tanks by air. Big Mouth lived another twelve years.This challenge was based on the Wangensteen approach with careful preoperative planning. This experience could also allow other facilities a record to use if whale surgery is necessary elsewhere in the world. The Minnesota influence again prevailed.

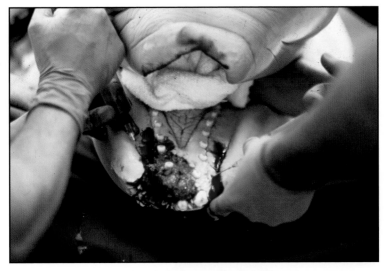

Local anesthesia prior to resection of mandible

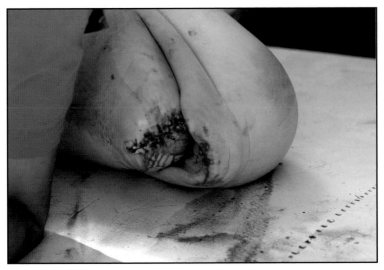

Post op after reconstruction

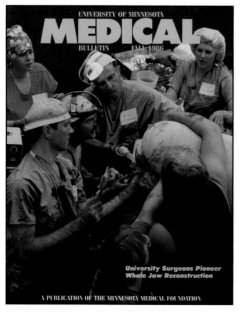

University Surgeons Pioneer Whale Jaw Reconstruction

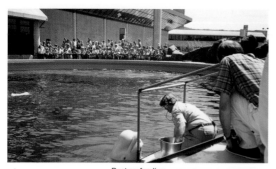

Post op feeding

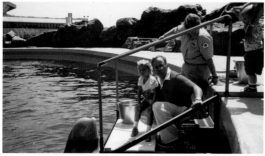

Dr. Leonard's weekly rounds with his grandchildren

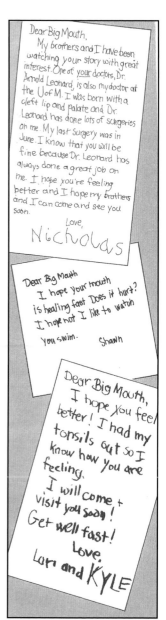

Dear Big Mouth,

My brothers and I have been watching your story with great interest. One of your doctors, Dr. Arnold Leonard, is also my doctor at the U of M. I was born with a cleft lip and palate and Dr. Leonard has done lots of surgeries on me. My last surgery was in June. I know that you will be fine because Dr. Leonard has always done a great job on me. I hope you're feeling better and I hope my brothers and I can come and see you soon.

Love,
Nicholas

Dear Big Mouth
I hope your mouth is healing fast Does it hurt? I hope not I like to watch you swim.   Shawn

Dear Big Mouth,
I hope you feel better! I had my tonsils out so I know how you are feeling.
I will come + visit you soon! Get well fast!
Love,
Lori and KYLE

Cards from children cheering on the whale

Chapter 15
Pediatric Surgery

Despite the early advances in cardiac pediatric surgery by Dr. C. Walton Lillehei, Dr. Richard Varco, Dr. Aldo Castaneda and Dr. Demetre Nicoloff, there was no pediatric intensive care and no area for pre-operation evaluation of pediatric patients. Wires from early pacemaker attempts were running everywhere. No pediatric intensivists (neonatologists) were full-time.

After being on Dr. Richard Varco's service and finishing my residency, I was asked, by Dr. Varco, if I could get the credentials to start a pediatric surgery division by spending a year with Dr. William Clatworthy in Columbus, Ohio at the Children's Hospital. Dr. Najarian and Dr. Wangensteen were very supportive. I left my family and traveled every two weeks from Columbus to Minneapolis and with support from the pediatric department, helped build an intensive care unit for infants and small children.

I also testified before the United States Congress regarding the necessity of specialized facilities and transportation support to decrease infant mortality in the United States, especially in areas such as Minnesota where rural specialized medical facilities were not available and the infant mortality was higher than most European countries. I also testified before the Minnesota Senate and received $80,000 for a "fly-in service". This fly-in program was instituted upon my return from Columbus as was our new neonatal and children's intensive care wards. This combination gave us the means of immediate implementation of a pediatric surgery division at the University of Minnesota with myself as chief of service.

The pediatric department was delighted and we began accepting and transporting patients with difficult problems who were losing their lives for lack of facilities in remote areas. A computerized monitoring system was eventually put in place, and integration of services begun. This program was a great advantage to the cardiac and later transplant services. I would initially fly out to pick up babies using a small bassinette heated with a heating pad. Intubation and intravenous therapy most frequently had to be instituted before transport. Our service grew rapidly and we thus, had one of the first fly-in service and computerized intensive care wards in the country.

We also participated with the children's tumor group in national studies. I designed the double lumen catheter and eventually the double port for combined chemotherapy and intravenous drugs, nutrition and fluid administration. This was necessary in the bone marrow transplant service and for large tumor problems. We combined our tumor treatment systems nationally and locally.

One of the most significant problems was large tumors in the liver, kidney and adrenal glands (neuroblastoma) as well as bone tumors such as osteogenic sarcoma, and muscle tumors (rhabdomyosarcomas). National randomized prospective studies were very helpful in the treatment of these problems, yet mortality and quality of life were constant issues. Neuroblastoma of adrenal origin stimulated us to embark in a new direction for tumor treatment, that of genetic engineering using the immune system as a basis for stimulation.

Dr. Dan Saltzman came into my laboratory and took on the challenge. He received his Ph.D. by doing original work of genetically engineering the salmonella organism with a human Interleukin 2 gene. We placed a second gene to detoxify the salmonella organism and if it reactivated, it would die. The salmonella was the vehicle used to travel to the liver, spleen, lungs, lymph nodes, stimulating the NK cells (natural killer lymphocytes) and T8 or cytotoxic lymphocytes to kill the cancers. A third (immunoflorescent) gene demonstrated the system also went directly to the liver and tumor. After 3,000 experiments over several years, FDA approval was granted and we are at present finishing Phase One trials. This is the first oral genetically engineered cancer drug approved. Most importantly by this technique in the laboratory, we were able to significantly reduce neuroblastoma as well as colon cancer and osteogenic sarcoma, one of the most lethal bone tumors of teenagers.

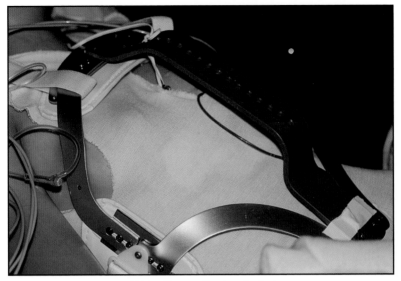

Pectus Brace with wire attached

At present, we are working to delineate the proteins and genes which stimulate tumor growth and those which aid tumor reduction. We will add the reduction complex and block the tumor growth complex to our present construct. This is the first generation of immune stimulation by an organism genetically engineered to kill tumor and can be given orally without complications. This is in contrast to chemotherapy. Quality of life is preserved. Our lab heads Brent Sorenson and Lance Augustin have been responsible for completing these studies and for ongoing research.

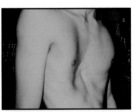

Pectus Excavatum deformity

Another problem which interested me was chest deformities. The operations to correct them seemed quite complicated, painful and moreover, generated expensive hospital stays. Thus, we devised an anterior one day procedure, correcting the deformity without undue thoracic intervention (opening the chest). We applied a brace post operatively which held a wire that had been previously

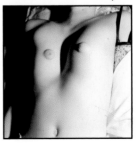

Pectus Excavatum deformity

104

operatively placed beneath the sternum to hold the sternum bone in place until healing occurred by a twelve week period. This new approach proved in a large number of patients to be efficient, gave a better quality of life, and was less expensive than the more invasive methods. Time will be the arbitrator.

Another important condition that needed correction of preoperative and postoperative routines was that of cystic fibrosis. Dr. Warren Warwick and I teamed up to clinically evaluate these children before and after correction of their surgical problems. Prior to this period, mortality and morbidity was high resulting in poor quality of life. Dr. Warwick demonstrated persistence and imagination in defining and designing testing apparatuses for pulmonary function (lung) and applied these concepts to patients before operative procedures.

Dr. Warwick also helped design a vest system to replace pummeling of the chest to relieve tenacious secretions. This procedure alone provided marked quality of life to these unfortunate patients. The application of evaluation parameters and correction of lung function, before and after surgical intervention, significantly reduced complications attributed to stress and anesthesia during these procedures. Today, these principles are also applied to adult patients with chronic obstructive lung disease and post operative chest trauma patients.

The vest system was funded by an Italian family who we were called to treat after a near cardiac arrest during surgery in Italy. After accepting the patient, we applied the principles established for cystic fibrosis. The patient survived for several years and lived in Minneapolis for the majority of her remaining life. The family, after I told them no charges were to be assessed because of the huge expense they endured, stated they were royalty and should be charged. I asked them, instead, to contribute to our research program in cystic fibrosis, especially in the testing of the vest technique. They contributed one million dollars toward a Chair in Cystic Fibrosis for ongoing correction of lung abnormalities. The Chair is properly held by Dr. Warren Warwick who has contributed so much in this field.

Through The Portals of Pigs and Manure

Dr. Saltzman has carried on his routine in the surgical area of this disease. The established principles and studies are used throughout the United States and the world. Interestingly enough I met Dan Saltzman in the early 1980's in Panama. He was twelve years old. I gave a lecture at the University of Panama on my newly innovative approaches to anterior spine surgery for scoliosis, degenerative and trauma problems. These operative procedures were carried out behind the peritoneum, in the pelvis, and thoracoabdominal (through the chest and abdomen). Dan's father ran the Panama Canal locks as an engineer and manufactured his own parts for lock problems. Dan asked me what I did and I explained the service at dinner in Dan's home. He said, "I want to do what you do." After his high school graduation, I got a call. He came to Minneapolis and completed his University pre-medical education followed by surgery residency. During his training, he did original work in genetic engineering in my lab and received his Ph.D. He subsequently received two years of pediatric surgery training. At present, he holds the Arnold S. Leonard, M.D., Ph.D. Endowed Chair in Pediatric Surgery, runs our research lab and has become Chief of Pediatric Surgery at the University of Minnesota. What better legacy knowing my surgery service is in such capable hands? The Wangensteen tradition continues.

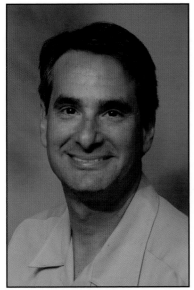

Dr. Daniel Saltzman

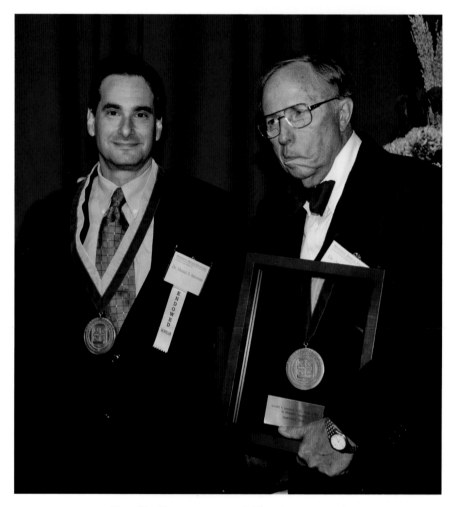

Dr. Saltzman and Dr. Leonard,
Endowed Chair Ceremony

Chapter 16
Conclusion

In conclusion, the Minnesota influence on American surgery is of a wide spectrum and subsequently diversifies to several important fields. The two major leaders, Dr. Owen Wangensteen and Dr. John Najarian are from different backgrounds and primary interests. However, they both are and were great teachers with similar philosophies. They transferred their own energies, intellectual powers, determination, imagination, and goal setting abilities to their students, who in turn produced many of the medical breakthroughs. Their persistence was of prime importance. These concepts of teacher influences are present in all educational levels from children to adults. They bring out the abilities of all pupils to query the unknown, and think beyond their dreams. All humans have this inert potential. Qualified, stimulating teachers must unearth this potential. These "Professors" of the human mind pass their qualities on to their fledglings and so on and so on and so on. How important these educators are, especially when schools and Universities present opportunities to become the paymasters of their lives. These individuals had great faith in young people and in education as a concept. Moreover, these advisors tapped the resources of potential creativity by sparking enthusiasm from their own examples. The greatness of these "mentors" are not measured by their own accomplishments, but by their continuous impact on those they have influenced. These individuals will, in turn, pass these precepts on to those who they influence, innovating new processes. As Carlyle best expressed it, "The lightning spark of thought generated in the solitary mind awaits its expressed likeness in another mind and a thousand other minds all blaze up together in a combined fire, the domino effect." All educational institutions should provide the fertile soil where critical masses of individuals can inter-relate, share ideas, and provide the basis for intellectual curiosity. It has been a privilege to spend most of my professional life in this prolific Minnesota academic community which has contributed so much to the history of American surgery.

Acknowledgements

Thank you to Dr. Wangensteen and his wife Sarah for the many weekly interviews, personal photos and notes prior to Dr. Wangensteen's retirement. Thanks also goes to the archives at the University of Minnesota and Jerry Vincent for many photos, to the many past residents, professors and visitors for their interviews over the past fifty years, and to Bonnie Har for her assistance in compiling these stories. I also thank John Najarian and Seldon Vickers for their continued support of our academic program, to Medtronic, and past CEO Earl Bakken, as well as Dr. Walt Lillehei, Dr. Clarence Dennis, Dr. Richard Varco, Dr. Edwards, and Dr. James Moller and their families for their interviews, personal histories, photos and notes. I also thank Tom and Jenny Arnfelt for their editorial comments. I extend much gratitude to Rob Evans and Michele Eichler for their efforts which have successfully raised funds for our genetic engineering research projects through the hunting industry, to Deana Peitz for her art renderings, and to the Carlson Print Group for their generous support of this project.

Reference Books

The Great American Surgical Training Centers and Surgical Mentors of the 20th Century by Leonard Peltier, M.D., Ph.D., and J. Bradley Aust, M.D., Ph.D., PUT. Publisher (family) 2009

The Rise of Surgery From Empirical Craft to Scientific Discipline by Owen H. Wangensteen and Sarah D. Wangensteen, 1978 University of Minnesota Press

Reflections of the Retiring Chief by Arnold S. Leonard, M.D., Ph.D., 1930-1967 University of Minnesota Press 1967

The Miracle of Transplantation, The Unique Odyssey of a Pioneer Surgeon by John S. Najarian, 2009 Phoenix Books Inc.

One Man's Full Life by Earl E. Bakken, 1999 Medtronic, Inc.

Machines in Our Hearts, The Cardiac Pacemaker, The Implantable Defibrillator, and American Health Care by Kirk Jeffrey, 2001 John Hopkins Press

Jesse E. Edwards, His Legacy to Cardiovascular Medicine by Brooks S. Edwards and James H. Moller, 2011 Science International Corp.

The Chief, Owen H. Wangensteen by Arnold S. Leonard, M.D., Ph.D., Medical Bulletin of Minnesota, Spring 1978

About the Author

Dr. Leonard, a Minnesota-born and worldwide medical pioneer, has been a surgeon specializing in orthopedic anterior spine approaches, thoracic surgery, general surgery, and pediatric surgery from 1956 to 2006. He has distinguished himself in a great number of areas. He was Head of Pediatric Surgery at the University of Minnesota from 1966-2004, and had membership in thirteen medical societies; receiving many special honors and awards including The Wangensteen Distinguished Professor Award for Excellence in Teaching; Lifetime Achievement Award from the Minnesota Medical Foundation, University of Minnesota Pediatric Surgery Department, and the University of Minnesota Amplatz Children's Hospital. He also received the Alumni Philanthropy and Service Award, honoring significant medical and philanthropic contributions to the Medical School, The University, and the community from the Minnesota Medical Foundation and the University of Minnesota Alumni Association. He is a member of several hospital and national medical committees; lecturer and author of over 270 abstracts, publications and presentations. He has also performed several research projects in the treatment of cancer, using genetic engineering to boost the immune system. He also performed the first whale surgery in the world. In 2004 the Arnold S. Leonard, M.D., Ph.D. Chair in Pediatric Surgery was awarded to Dr. Leonard by the University of Minnesota as an endowed scholar, along with other distinguished surgery department Minnesota physicians. This is one of the highest honors given by the University of Minnesota. Also an endowed lectureship in pediatric surgery in his name was awarded to Dr. Leonard by the Department of Surgery at the University of Minnesota in 2010.